Bharat S. Shah, M.D. presents

Questions, Answers, and Exclamations

From the Garage of a Clinical Researcher

Setubandh Publications
New York

Questions, Answers, and Exclamations
From the Garage of a Clinical Researcher
By Bharat S. Shah, M.D.

ISBN #   13:978-1456589349
           10:   1456589342

First U.S. Edition 2011

U.S. $15.00

Please see the end pages for other books by the author

This book is

dedicated to all my teachers, like

Dr. V. S. Ajgaonkar, Late Dr. T. H. Rindani,

(of Topiwala National Medical College, Mumbai)

Late Mr. G. H. Jambotkar, Late Mr. Jayant C. Shah,

(of Babu Panalal P. Jain High School, Mumbai)

Late Lothar Wertheimer, M.D.

(Of New York Medical College, New York)

and many others from whom

I have learned formally and informally,

in person or across the great divide of time and place,

and whom I can only hope to emulate by

calling myself a Doctor ("a teacher")

❖

कालोऽयं च निरवधि विपुला च पृथ्वी ।   (उत्तररामचरिते भवभूति)

The time is endless
The Earth is boundless!   *(Bhvabhuti in the UttarRamCharitum)*

(Someday, someone, somewhere will appreciate this!)

PREFACE

"The art is long and the life is short!" The father of medicine, Hippocrates said it long time ago. We do know that the art of medicine is endless and our own life is short, we do not know how short. In that short life one can accumulate enough debt to the society, which has to be paid back before one departs — even though one may not be in any hurry to do that.

A research worker fascinated by life, gathers innumerable ideas, undertakes numerous projects, completes a few of them, drops a few, reaches several dead ends, and collects a drawerful of rejections of his or her works.

Medical journals are not in the business of doling out praise and appreciation, or to admire the effort that goes into a research project from its inception through publication. They have their own standards for selecting the papers to publish. They also have to assess the idea, the approach, the study design, methods, analyses-statistical and otherwise, validity of the conclusions drawn, plus sophistication and interest of its readers.

All these are valid and essential to serve some purpose. However, a research worker can stomach only so many rejections. After all, (s)he is also a human being, even though it may not seem so at times. Just as some love can blossom after the marriage, some peer reviews can take place after publication, as was the standard practice in the days of Einstein, Newton, Galen, Maimonides, Charak, and Sushrut.

Not all researchers have enough time left to wait till they get the Nobel prize, when they can publicly display all rejection slips from prestigious journals. In most cases the ideas would simply die with the researcher. They become extinct and as is said quite well, "The extinction is for ever!"

We cannot afford it. Therefore, with utmost respect for the age old and time honored traditions, with no intention of bypassing them, I undertake this self publication of all my research ideas and bequeath them to the posterity. Let someone else amend them and carry them to their fruition. Rather than bypassing a peer review, I am again submitting to it. Unlike submission, ideas should not be rejected.

I have been a clinician taking care of patients. Doing research work was never in my job description, and most of my research work was carried out in hospitals that were not primarily involved in research, or where research was often a dirty word generating a hostile response.

All these ideas and projects had been reviewed and approved by appropriate committees as required by regulations of that time. They are presented here in an interesting and simple narration *for even a lay person to understand*. We never know who may pick them up. Maybe, it can attract someone to our profession.

I have no qualms, resentment, gripe, or grievances against any aspect of medical publishing. There is always some room for improvement. I believe that the medical publishing has not taken enough advantage of the great revolution in the individual freedom that the desk-top-publishing and on-demand-printing have heralded. Our thinking needs to be adjusted and fine tuned in that regard.

There should be nothing against self publishing. An author has to stand up behind his or her work. However, one cannot wait until everybody else gets behind it as well. That may take several life times and yet, the work may not be appreciated. Publishing saves it from getting perished, even after the researcher does so. Saving ideas may not be any less important than saving a life.

In the part: I of the book, I have presented the ideas, how they came about, how they were developed, executed and introduced into practice, what blocked them, what role did the luck, accident and serendipity play in their progress, and the how much fascination and frustration they generated along the way.

I have also pointed out what still remains to be done and what can be done in the future to open up the idea for other applications, wherever I could see far enough. Technical details have been kept to a minimum in this part. Hardly any data are presented, except when they are absolutely necessary to make the point clear.

The part: II contains most of my unpublished research papers and articles as such, *current as of the date they were last amended*, with Abstract, Introduction, Materials and Methods, Observations and Results, and Discussion sections, followed by Bibliography. This will be better appreciated by those who prefer to look at papers presented methodically in that order. Future researchers would have to bring these to the standards prevailing in their times.

Papers in the part: II are not presented here for the reader to judge whether the journals were justified in rejecting them. I am sure they were. That is not the point now. What is intended is for someone to get the idea, develop it properly or differently and make it work for maybe another purpose. I hope to generate the proverbial light, not heat.

Almost all projects have been my works, with some people helping me get them published by a particular organization requiring its membership as a precondition for submission. Some of my department heads have refrained from adding their names as co-authors despite their significant help.

As for the acknowledgements, I would be at a complete loss about where to begin and whom to include. At every step, I have been fortunate to have had support from innumerable people and sources, to all of whom I am deeply indebted. I cannot forget my experimental animals, human volunteers, staff of various labs, family and friends, professional mentors and those people whose contributions I am not even aware of.

Before I got my own balls (typing elements for the IBM Selectric typewriter, that is) and started doing my own typing, most of the papers in this work were meticulously typed over and over, maybe 5-6 times each, as demanded by various journals, by Ms. Maxine Helffrick, our secretary in the Department of Medicine at the Coler Memorial Hospital.

One thing I cannot be accused of is, sitting on my results rather than sending them out for publication. Although I have not been hungry for publication, promotion, grant money, tenure, etc., maybe, because they were not going to come my way in the para-academic track, I have shared my results with anybody and everybody who would care to listen, or at least appear to do so and often, not even that.

What would I say to the future research worker? Well, keep working, and always respect and enjoy the wonder and the miracle that is life. All other rewards may or may not come, most likely they would not. Therefore, if you do not enjoy the research in itself, don't torment yourself and your family by being in it.

They say, "You plant the trees for the posterity." I would say, you plan projects also for the posterity. That is the only way you can pay back your debt to your ancestors, on whose giant shoulders you stood to look in the distance, into the *terra incognita!*

Bharat S. Shah, M.D.
New York.
<bharatkumarshah@pol.net>
October 2, 2011.

TABLE OF CONTENTS

PART: II
REJECTIONS' HALL OF FAME!

✸✸✸

QUESTIONS,

ANSWERS,

AND

EXCLAMATIONS

FROM THE GARAGE OF A CLINICAL RESEARCHER

PART: I

IDEAS, YOURS FOR ASKING!

1. INTRODUCTION

Every mother knows that her infant son or daughter is destined to be the future President of the United States, or its equivalent in other countries. Every research worker is sure of becoming a Nobel laureate someday. These expectations are reasonable and, despite the infinitesimal chance of their fulfillment understandable. What is overlooked by a casual observer is the amount of hard work, devotion and love that goes into their pursuit.

Although one may enjoy it, the pursuit is indeed that of apparent unhappiness. It is venturing into the unknown territory which makes it fascinating and scary. It is easy to understand the preceding intellectually, but not emotionally. Research may represent prestige, maybe money, maybe fame, maybe a promotion, maybe a Nobel prize, but foremost, it is a rebellion, or a counter revolution in some cases.

There are several kinds of medical research workers. Some may try to explore the limits of established ideas, confirm findings of other workers, or try to refute them. Some may have a machine to measure something and use it to make millions of observations over a period and then attempt to find a new pattern therein. Some review all the work done to date and synthesize it into a new framework. All these are important. Then there is the researcher who starts with new ideas, new explanations, new devices and new applications of existing material in a creative way.

To an extent all research can be said to begin with an idea, because there is something that bothers the researcher about something that (s)he has noticed. It does not fit with what is known, or believed to be true. The researcher has to investigate the issue and may find that the conventional thinking is either inadequate, mistaken, or dead wrong. This is where the rebellion comes in the picture.

(S)he is the "wise guy," who now knows better than everybody else who is quite happily working without any problem with the idea as interpreted that far. Are all of them fools? Are they blind? What about all their work? Is it now meaningless? It is the researcher against the rest of the world, the entire globe, going back to the beginning of that idea. Try to imagine that you have inferred from your observations that the earth is indeed flat! This rebellion is to be fought single-handedly. That is intimidating enough.

What is more frightening is, mother nature has chosen him over everybody else, to reveal her secrets and she is standing stark naked in front of him. As if the worker has just concluded that the President is a spy for a foreign country!

Even if (s)he can prove to himself or herself that (s)he is correct and the old interpretation is incorrect, that is not the end of it. He has to appease others that they are neither fools nor lost, and *that there is an explanation why the old interpretation came about*. This aspect, stressed by Karl Popper in his masterpiece, "The Logic of Scientific Discovery," is ignored by many researchers to their own peril.

Let me give one example. Say we are sitting at the dining table, sipping tea or coffee from your finest china and having wonderful time. Now, to show off my smartness, I can enlighten you that the dining table is made up of innumerable small particles called atoms. You will barely acknowledge my stating the obvious known to everybody.

Since you are not yet impressed, I go on to tell you that these atoms are made of a central nucleus, with several other particles called *electrons* orbiting it. In short, the table is anything but a solid stable structure capable of safely supporting your precious china. You hesitate to put your, by now empty cup on it.

Although according to me, now your world view is quite wrong, it is also as right as it has always had been. *This capacity to harbor two or more mutually exclusive notions simultaneously is a characteristic of a creative mind.*

Our view of the world and the cosmos is made of building blocks, somewhat like Legos. Scientists can arrange them every which way to suggest the structure of the whole, but that structure can be replaced by another more acceptable one, when the latter comes around.

Popper states in the same book, *"The best thing that can happen to a scientific theory is to be proved wrong, because that is how the science progresses."* The best thing that can happen to an acorn nut is to get wet and crack. That is how a new mighty oak tree can come to life. Pending that, the squirrel can merrily munch on it.

There are many books written on ideas, creativity, research, accidents, serendipity and what not. Therefore, I will not dwell on these. Of millions of people, only a few are in position to get struck by an idea, a paradox, something different, maybe upside down. Most of them would just walk away from it. That is the wise thing to do. Remember, it is not easy to live with it.

It is one's prerogative to walk away from an idea. One may refuse to let the idea enter one's mind. However, once an idea enters the mind, it just commandeers the latter. It takes complete control of it and does not let that person think of anything else. If this sounds like love, it is. This is what being possessed is all about. You cannot be possessed and be "normal" at the same time.

You, possessed by the idea, live in a different world now. You are pregnant with an idea, with the future President, or the Nobel prize winner. If you consider the odds of taking an idea to its fruition, you can begin to appreciate why an idea is precious. It is an important piece of the cosmic puzzle, an important piece of evidence to nail down a case. You cannot afford to ignore it, or neglect to nurture it. Well, unfortunately that is exactly what most of us do.

Some rare ones cannot. They are obsessed with being unhappy, not necessarily aware that someday their work may make others happy. Prestige, money, etc., are not visible even on the horizon yet. Only the work on hand, a mission of sorts, with no instruction manual or a design or even all parts of the puzzle, is staring you in the eyes.

I have always admired them and tried to emulate them. In my professional life as a practicing physician, I have stumbled upon several ideas, some practical, while others too esoteric to help my patients either directly, or through advancing the basic science.

Although it is love, "Till death do us part," is not an option. Not everything can be achieved in one life time. Being born in India, I probably have many more births and lives left, but I cannot entrust these ideas to my already vanishing memory to recall them in the next life.

When an American football player finds it impossible to carry the ball any further, he "passes" it to another teammate, rather than letting it die. *This is my last will and testament to bequeath my medical research ideas and projects to the posterity with the proviso that it will never let them be extinguished!*

2. THE WONDER OF SCIENCE

While reading some books on scientific discoveries and inventions, one gets the feeling as if one is reading the sports section of the Monday's newspaper. The race to the top or to be the first or to win the Nobel or another prize is the only thing that seems to matter. Major breakthroughs, hitting the pay dirt and being successful in producing positive results are applauded. Efforts and contributions of individuals or their groups are exalted. All this is good, as far as it goes.

What is lost in the excitement of the horse race or the rat race is the importance of searching for the truth, which is supposed to be the main, if not the sole purpose of scientific research. What is also forgotten is, contribution of or the groundwork done by the giants who antedated the present worker. Even though apparently being carried out in an isolated and maybe dilapidated lab or in a garage, research is still a collective pursuit.

Individuals come in the picture either as the ones who generate ideas, or develop them, or hold on to them, or nurture them and cling to them to carry them to their fruition. Most of these ideas and workers remain in oblivion, their role as birthplace of or foundation of all research remains all but invisible. That should not bother them and it does not, in most instances. They pursue the truth and their happiness comes from that pursuit.

Almost all books on research have been written by the most successful super achievers in the field, showing us how arduous their journey was rather than being a flash of miracle. It is good for ordinary mortals to know about their journey and try to emulate them. That ends up being an exercise in frustration and envy, reinforcing one's inferiority, rather than encouraging one to join the pursuit. Someone else's success is a poor motivator.

Determination and perseverance come later, experience comes from failure which comes only after one tries to do something. These do help in sustaining the research worker, who has to be hooked on to the research in first place. That hook is subconscious, more emotional than intellectual. It has to sweep one off one's feet, after which nothing matters. That feels wonderful.

Like other best things in the world, feeling of wonder is also free and hence not appreciated or embraced by many. Eyes blinded by glitter cannot see it, heart chasing the success has no room for it. Wonder lives in a child's wide open eyes and in a lover's heart.

The Indian goddess of success and wealth, *Laxmi* is quite well known in the West. The Greek goddess of love, *Aphrodite* is also known. In our western society blindly in love with wealth, it is understandable that the Indian muse of learning, *Saraswati* is not known that well.

Saraswati is a beautiful maiden, clad in a white *sari*, seated on the white lotus flower, carrying a string instrument, *Veena,* in her hand, with a peacock dancing nearby. She is the daughter of the creator aspect, the four-headed *Brahma*, is an eternal virgin and yet, is considered a mother, like Christ's mother, Mary. Engaging in research is pursuing Saraswati, neither Laxmi, nor Aphrodite.

A little explanation is in order here. In the western world, undergraduates are called *Bachelors* and they do what bachelors do the best—chasing enticing maidens and succeeding in that eventually to become their *Masters*. Then one can learn more and be able to teach that subject to others, after becoming a *Doctor of (that particular) Philosophy*.

I have met innumerable doctors, both, Ph.D. and M.D., but have not come across many who could tell me what the word *doctor* means. It means *teacher*, who teaches, studies and pursues knowledge. It has nothing to do with luxury cars, palatial dwellings, or golf courses.

According to the eastern philosophy, one cannot be the master of one's mother. Saraswati is beautiful, gorgeous and enticing. She lures you into the woods of the unknown. She enjoys it when you get lost, when she appears again, making you chase her. You always get the feeling that she is within your reach and would be in your arms any minute but, she is not to be held. She is an eternal virgin, pure white. If you could have her, then she would not be worth having! Pursuit is at least as much fun as success. This is what needs to be conveyed to all potential research workers.

Wonder probably cannot be imparted. Even when one shows a wonderful thing to another person, the latter may see it but may not feel the wonder. It is a very personal thing, maybe a gift, worth cultivating, at least worth nurturing by not killing the child within us.

In my childhood in Mumbai (Bombay then), we used to play on a relatively huge terrace on the sixth level from which one had a bird's eye view of the entire city. At both ends of the terrace, there were iron water tanks supported on foot high concrete blocks, leaving the area underneath them quite dark and wet from minor leaks and condensation of water. There was no shortage of dirt either.

The floor of the terrace was covered with layers of tar and black, sharp gravel which somehow never deterred our delicate feet from running on it. One day, I saw a small sprout raising its head from the mud near the edge of the bottom of the tanks. There were a few more saplings of different sizes.

That delicate, green seedling in dirty, smelly mud flat, on a harsh gravel floor had something in it to make the child that I was, identify with it. For the next few days, no trip to the terrace went without paying a visit to my that new friend. On picking it up, I saw two parts of a seed lifted above the ground, together with two tiny leaves cradling them.

A few years later, my father took us to the Kamala Nehru Park on the nearby Malabar Hills. My eyes were glued on the colorful coleus plants edging the flower beds. That was the first time ever that I saw a leaf of several colors. Green, red, chocolate, all on the same leaf. Flowers are colorful, but leaves, too!

Seeing plants and animals was nothing new for me. I was born in a village and we used to go there to spend our vacations. Village butchers would drag the carcasses of dead cows, water buffaloes and other animals to the outskirts, to skin and butcher them. My intense desire to go there and watch that dirty, smelly and most unhygienic scene was quite properly vetoed by my Jain vegetarian elders, for my own protection.

One can shelter a child from an open carcass, but not from the open sky. There was no electricity or running water in that village then and stray animals, snakes and scorpions were abundant. We were under strict admonition against leaving our foot high bed under the open sky without letting an elder know.

On a moonless night, my eyes opened in the middle of the night, thinking of calling an uncle or an aunt to take me to answer the nature's call. My mouth opened up for a different reason. The post-midnight sky was studded with innumerable bight stars of all sizes and brightness. There was a bright band of light stretching across the entire sky. It was not like what one sees in a planetarium. It was not a flat picture. The stars were at varying depths, too!

That was the first and the last time I saw the Milky Way, our own galaxy, spanning the whole sky. Later during my adult life, on night trips through the countryside, I have hoped to see the Milky Way, to no avail. Light can be more blinding than darkness. In the city lights, one can watch TV, but not the moon or the stars.

My primary, middle and secondary school years were enjoyable. Teachers, parents and others had not done anything to squash my curiosity, creativity, or sense of wonder. Exposure to literature, philosophy and religion had served to deepen those. We were not praised for every little thing. Even for big things done well, we were accustomed to hear, "Good, but...!" and that never bothered us.

Girls our age we were not supposed to talk to, sparing us the possible cruel humiliation engendered by their generous giggles. Grown up and recently married neighborhood young women, or daughters-in-law played with us and kept our life in quiet balance. Entire neighborhood was a vigilante system to prevent us from letting our curiosity take better of us and get involved with the street people.

In those days good students chose engineering or medicine after their high school. After the first or the freshman year in the science college, we had to choose between the two branches of science. I was comfortable with either, but was leaning towards engineering. "Freshman five" refers to the weight gain of that group. However, we lost that much.

The high school education was in Gujarati, our mother tongue, as the medium of instruction. We did study English as a subject during the middle and the high school years. That was mostly the written English, correct grammatically. To speak or understand the spoken English was impossible. Mathematics was not much dependent on the language, at least in writing. So that was a lucrative shelter.

If English was impossible, Biology was in Latin. Our friends and colleagues either kept mum in the class, or asked meanings of words like "penis," or "anus," being appreciated by the rest of us for doing that, while embarrassing the professors, who sometimes were kind enough to resort to local languages.

The sapling under the water tanks had been growing quietly and the coleus from the Kamala Nehru Park had acquired a few more hues. I saw the onion peel under the microscope and thought of the midnight sky with the Milky Way. Plants could eat small insects, animals could be immobile, what we thought to be fruits were roots and the other way around.

The design of various systems of reproduction, photosynthesis, defense, etc., was fantastic. The difference between the living and the nonliving, that between the plant cells and the animal ones was fascinating. The life forms sitting on the fence between those divisions, e.g., bacteria are more like plants than animals, viruses are between living and nonliving were mysterious. Life was taking hold of us.

We are also parts of that animal kingdom and our own growing bodies also were coming to life in a strange and pleasant way. After the sexual segregation of neighborhood and the school years, the college was co-educational. Presence of girls or young women around us was pleasantly disturbing.

The atmosphere in my college was extremely serious and was sexually not charged at all. Biology was attracting me only in the abstract, without any individual attachment, without my eyes lusting after any particular part of the soft company around me. We were just slightly beyond the birds and bees.

We did not have the venerable National Geographic magazine there, with women in their natural attire or the lack of it. A friend of mine showed me a photograph of two grasshoppers in mating, then both of us went on to find similar illustrations in that book and in others. The life was sweeping me off my feet.

I found myself spending more time studying biology than sharpening the maths. As it is, biology demanded more time, since it was not a point scoring subject and its terminology was Latin—with little obvious similarity with any of the Indian languages. Come what may, biology was the way to go. Good bye, mathematics. I will miss you!

I stopped devoting any time to the maths, confident that I knew enough of it to clear the exam. In biology, my grades were understandably not as good, but they would have to get better. Without any formal teaching of Latin, I extracted on my own, some rules governing it. Soon, I began to feel comfortable with it and saw my command over English also getting better.

The technical terms in medicine are Greek, literally. My knowledge of Latin prefixes and suffixes was applied to decipher those of the Greek language, with good outcome. Many terms depended heavily on the rich Greek mythology, learning which was fun, painful though it was. After studying the basic sciences, namely, anatomy and physiology in the med school, I ventured into the clinical medicine, where the real patients are!

3. TEMPERATURE AND HEART RATE

In India, medical schools are called "colleges," and their years are each 18 months long. We had to complete three such "years" of study and then do a 12 month long *rotating internship* in various departments before obtaining our MBBS (Bachelor of Medicine and Surgery) degree. First MBBS was devoted to studying Anatomy and Physiology.

Second and third years are called *clinical years* because that is when students study Medicine and Surgery and are exposed to various subspecialties. Second year is exciting, confusing and frightening. In the beginning of that year, students are thoroughly lost. They know the human anatomy and physiology, but have not developed the judgement what a normal body is really like.

They start studying the abnormal body, or the pathology. They may be studying the heart in the classrooms and how to examine the lungs, on the wards. Demonstrations and tutorials may deal with still something else. Maybe, not intended to be confusing, this system does familiarize the future doctors with a chaotic life lying ahead.

Learning to examine the living human bodies, both male and female, is far from confusing or chaotic. After dealing with formalin soaked and ice cold cadavers, it is a pleasant relief to touch the breathing human beings. Assessing the vital signs is the first thing to learn. Temperature, pulse and respiration or *TPR* in short, constitute the *vital signs* that doctors rely on to assess their patients. They provide an idea of general condition of the patient.

Before any fancy instruments became available, doctors held hands of their patients and took the pulse. They studied its rhythm, force, etc. and got a general idea of whether it was too fast or too slow. This method of assessment is as old as medicine. Determining the precise pulse rate had to wait for hundreds or thousands of years for a practical watch to be invented in the seventeenth century.

Similarly, doctors had to physically feel patient's forehead to see whether it was too hot, or too cold. Precise measurement of body temperature had to await the arrival of a practical portable thermometer on the scene around 1860s.

Pulse rate varies from moment to moment and is affected by many factors. Physiological or "normal" entities like anxiety, excitement, arousal, fear, exercise, age, all affect pulse rate. Then there are innumerable disease conditions of heart and other organs, known as "pathological causes" which can alter the pulse rate.

Relationship of body temperature and pulse rate is the first one that a student learns in *physical diagnosis*. The latter is the art and science of trying to reach a diagnosis using only physical examination, without any lab tests, EKG, Xray and other entities. Taking a detailed history from patient precedes laying a hand on him or her. More than half of the diagnoses can be arrived at by taking the proper history alone.

History and physical examination can help the doctor reach a diagnosis in up to 80% of his patients. other technological tools may or may not be always available, but one's sense organs are always there. Even in countries with advanced medical care, emergencies occurring on highways or in remote mountains may test a doctor's skills in physical diagnosis.

No matter how variable patients' pulse rate is, it bears a stable relation with body temperature. An increase in body temperature is associated with a rise in pulse rate or heart rate, the latter terms are usually interchangeable under most conditions. Determining the heart rate requires listening to the heart with a stethoscope.

To state the rule more precisely, *every change in body temperature by one degree Celsius, is accompanied by that in the mean pulse rate by ten beats per minute.* That is, if pulse rate is 70 beats/min at body temperature 37 °C (approximately 98 °F), it is expected to be 80/min, if the temperature increases to 38 °C. At 40 °C, pulse goes up to 100/min.

Pulse rate is not called *mean* to describe its personality. *Mean* signifies an average of several readings, since pulse rate is so variable from moment to moment. There are conditions like typhoid fever in which the change in pulse rate is less striking, that is, instead of going up by 10 beats, it may do so by say 4-5 beats. Typhoid fever of 40 °C may be associated with only 80/min pulse rate, rather than the expected 100/min.

It should be noted that 80/min is still more than 70/min, in other words, it is still a faster rate, but is slower than what one would expect. So, typhoid fever is associated with a *relatively* slow rate. The technical Greek word for fast is *Tachy* and for slow is *Brady*. Therefore, in typhoid, we see a *relative bradycardia* or a slower than expected hear rate. Presence of this sign alone may clinch the diagnosis of typhoid fever. Who says medicine is difficult!

Well, it is not difficult. However, your students can always make your life difficult. When our instructor in Physical Diagnosis, Dr. Ajgaonkar taught us this rule describing the temperature-pulse relationship and mentioned the exception of typhoid fever, I raised my hand to ask, why? He left the podium, walked slowly towards me, put his one hand on my shoulder and said, "That's for you to find out!"

"Who me?" I did not say that out loud, but looked at him nodding to say *yes.* He continued,

"Medicine has come a long way, but not everything is known or understood yet." He could have fooled me. There I was, sitting and worrying that everything was already discovered and I was there to get all of it from him and other professors! After all, there was something left for me to do. I looked up at him, as if to say,

"Why not? With your blessings, you never know!"

4. DOES ANYBODY FOLLOW THE RULE?

After completing the internship and earning my MBBS degree, I prepared the necessary documents to come to the U.S.A. In New York State, internship is done after getting the M.D., therefore, I had to repeat the internship. Then I joined a residency program in Internal Medicine.

Keeping of medical records is a sacred activity carried out diligently—often too diligently, as I was to find out much later—by doctors and hospitals. Nurses record the vital signs several times a day, as ordered by doctors. Temperature and pulse rate are graphically recorded, or "charted" at least once daily. Sicker patients and those in the intensive care units are observed more thoroughly.

The hospital in New York where I did my Medicine residency, and its affiliated hospitals were short stay *acute care* facilities, where patients were admitted for a few days or maybe a week or two and were discharged, while a few of them died. I do not quite know why, but I had begun to look at the temperature-pulse records more carefully than what was needed.

Maybe, I had spotted one or two instances where the temperature-pulse relationship was at odds with what I had studied. Boredom of repeating the internship may have made my mind wander for some stimulation.

The above practice soon became a routine, almost an obsession. To make proper and meaningful observation, sizable number of data points should be looked at. other than in the ICUs, data recording was sketchy, with lot of missing points. ICU records were better, but pulse rate in very week patients can change substantially on slightest exertion, unrelated to body temperature.

Every now and then, I found sufficiently long stretch of available data points. Hospital vital signs are charted on a graph paper. Levels of temperature and pulse rate are plotted on the two vertical (Y) axes and the time of the record on the horizontal (X) axis.

The scales are adjusted to make the temperature and corresponding expected heart rate fall close by, e.g., 98.6 °F and 70/min will share the same location on the vertical axes. The rest of the graph shows higher and lower temperatures and corresponding heart rates. Any deviant pattern would be immediately noticeable.

Temperature is generally plotted using the blue or black ink pen and heart rate is plotted in red. If the red line is above the darker one, that indicates a relatively rapid heart and if it is lower, then the heart is slower. Both these variations can occur for many reasons, and were seen by me in many records.

Typhoid fever would produce the pattern of red line below the blue or black one indicating a relative bradycardia or slower heart. Typhoid is a rare condition to be seen in hospitals in the U.S. It should be recalled that typhoid fever is only a variant of temperature-pulse relationship; a rise in temperature is still associated with an increase in the pulse rate, albeit, to a lesser extent.

At times I noticed temperature and pulse rate going their own way, rather than remaining in tandem. I had never seen or heard about such a phenomenon before. Now on, we will use the following abbreviations:

BT   for body temperature
PR   for pulse rate.

We will also use the following abbreviations:

TP-S   The conventional relationship wherein body temperature (BT), and pulse (PR) both go in the *same* direction,

TP-OP   BT and PR moving in *opposite* directions

TP-Z   BT or PR showing no (*zero*) or insignificant change.

In many patients, on some days when body temperature increased, pulse rate decreased and the other way around (TP-OP). This did not occur all the time on the same day. If vital signs were taken eight times in a day, various combinations of TP-S, TP-OP and TP-Z occurred say, 2-2-3 times, respectively, during the seven time slots.

When a patient goes into *the shock,* or a circulatory collapse, the skin becomes cold because of poor circulation and pulse gets faster in an attempt to help it pick up. This is TP-OP, but it is a one time event. Shock does not occur repeatedly. What I saw was frequent reversals in which temperature may increase or decrease and pulse may behave in the opposite manner.

In many instances, TP-OP completely replaced TP-S for hours and days on end. That was strange. TP-S was ingrained in our minds as the standard BT-PR behavior expressed as a codified rule. Was it possible that the rule supposedly applied only to people who are not sick or hospitalized? It did not seem so. We were not taught that rule in our

physiology lectures during the first MBBS. We were introduced to it as a prelude to our entry into the hospital.

It is common for almost any rule to have a few exceptions. What I was witnessing was sheer chaos! Was the rule
valid at all, or was I looking at the proverbial Chinese Emperor's clothes?

5. DIAMONDS
ARE THEY GIRLS' BEST FRIENDS?

Graphic records of vital signs have been receiving less and less attention in modern hospitals. There are far more sophisticated and specific tests to help doctors make a diagnosis. When they are looked at, it is generally to see whether a patient has been running a fever. Heart rate record is rarely paid attention to and relationship between the two is just never looked at.

Once in our class in Topiwala National Medical College, Mumbai, Dr. Ajgaonkar asked us to state our hobbies. My answer was, "To pay attention to every little apparently insignificant things that no one else is interested in." So, it must have started long before that, I suppose. I won't take any questions about this quirk of my personality. I simply do not know what else to say.

During the next two years after my internship and Medicine residency, I was at the Manhattan V. A. Hospital in New York City, where many patients were ambulatory and their vital signs were recorded infrequently. In those days before the belt tightening came to medicine, hospitals were in no hurry to discharge patients to the community. There was no ulterior motive involved.

We will return to the V. A. Hospital in New York City, where I did my fellowship in diseases of the chest, or Pulmonary Medicine, later on to spend lot more time there. For now, let us move on.

After completing residency and fellowship, I became a licensed physician and started working at the Coler Memorial Hospital operated by New York's Health and Hospitals Corporation (HHC). It was a long term or chronic care facility, where patients with intractable diseases spent months and years of their lives. It was a 1600 bed hospital and was to become a 450 bed nursing home and hospital over the next decade, first of almost two that I was going to spend there.

It had its own equivalent of a lower level ICU, called an Acute Care Unit or ACU, where sicker patients not requiring an outside hospital referral were treated. They stayed in the unit for weeks and months. Nursing staff recorded their temperature and heart rate every four hours and plotted them meticulously. Doctors looked at these records only slightly more frequently than in other facilities. Maybe, that was a ploy of the goddess Saraswati to lure me into it, in her usual way. I was her willing and eager prey.

Before going further, let me get a few cliches out of the way. Any new discovery has to suffer through stereotype responses in stages. First there is disbelief, "It cannot be! If it was there, we would have seen it." That puts the data under suspicion. "Well, you cannot rely on the data gathered from patients' charts. Their recording is so poor! Have you seen the way these nurses and nurses' aides take temperature?"

Then the value of the findings is questioned. "It is probably an artifact," or "Even if it is true, so what? It is not going to be of any use to anybody anyway!" The final blow comes—"Do you think everybody all over the world and through the entire history has been a fool and you are the wisest one to show that what they have been doing is all for nothing?"

In extreme cases, a researcher may be burned at stakes, or be excommunicated. Throughout this book, we will see repeatedly that none of these problems plagued me. You will have to wait for the appropriate moment to know that. I have always had a soft corner for the nurses and their assistants. Even in modern times, they work like slaves and hand maidens of doctors and other authority figures in the hospital. I was yet to see up close their devotion and love for the patients who could not even thank them.

Let us assume for the sake of the argument that the phenomenon of TP-OP was an artifact created entirely by sloppy data gathering followed by equally irresponsible charting. The question still remains, what would anyone gain from perpetrating such a hoax? Since hardly anybody bothered to look at that—the nurses' magnificent art work— why would they even do that and how?

In any research, medical or otherwise, when any new observation is made, before going into its possible impor- tance, one has to rule out the possibility of its being a chance or a random event. There are other pitfalls, too. Data have (the noun "data" is always plural) to be free from bias of all kinds. For example, how likely is it for you to see all seven trucks to belong to the UPS? Very much so, if you are stand- ing in its warehouse parking lot!

There are statistical tests to rule out such eventuali- ties. At this juncture, please remove from your minds sum- marily, all defamations and belittling jokes about the statis- tics and its methods. It is only a tool to help an observer de- termine with some degree of confidence, whether his or her data can be explained away as a chance event. One may think that it may be extremely rare for a coin to land head up six out six times. However, if you repeat that experiment

100 times, of six tosses each, you can get six heads out of six, more than five times.

To state that in scientific terms, there is a 5% chance for one to get all six heads in six coin tosses. Seven out of seven is borderline, just short of becoming significant at 5% level and eight of eight is significant at 5% level. Even though eight out of eight heads is possible less than 5% of the times, it is nonetheless possible. In medical research, 5% possibility of data being caused by a chance event is accepted as being significant. In the technical lingo,

The data were statistically significant at 5% level, or

The *"p" value* (probability of its being a chance)
was less than .05, or

$p \leq 5\%$, or

$p \leq 0.05$.

I would urge the reader to go over the above a few times and understand it well before going on. The above assessment of significance is only a statistical index, having nothing to do with the real life importance of anything. Even one murder in a population of ten million people is significant on any day. On the contrary, a minor or trivial change in a large number of population may be statistically significant, but may have no relevance otherwise.

***

	BT Increased	BT Decreased	BT Unchanged
PR Increased	TP-S	TP-OP	TP-Z
PR Decreased	TP-OP	TP-S	TP-Z
PR Unchanged	TP-Z	TP-Z	TP-Z

Table: 1. Various possible combinations and permutations of BT and PR. Note that there are two TP-S, two TP-OP and five TP-Z.

As shown in the above table, during any time slot BT may either increase, decrease, or remain unchanged. Similarly PR can do the same. Thus there are nine possible permutations and combinations of BT and PR relationship. In two of them BP and PR both may increase or may both decrease (TP-S). In other two, one may increase while the other decreases (TP-OP). In two more each, BT or PR may remain unchanged and in one more, both may remain unchanged.

Thus conventional TP-S by chance alone can occur two of nine times, as can TP-OP. The TP-Z is overwhelmingly more likely to occur by chance alone five out of nine times. If there were no particular relationship of BT and PR, *relative random frequencies* of various kinds of TPs by chance would be, 2, 2 and 5 out of total 9.

When I tabulated the frequencies of TP-OP and others, TP-OP was found to occur far more frequently than merely 2 out of 9 times and was significant at better than one percent level, or p < 0.01. I have spared you the actual numbers, because these findings were reported in a letter to the editor[1] of the Journal of the AMA.

Thus far, my interest was limited to showing that this newly observed strange TP-OP was a random event of no significance, but I ended up proving quite the opposite of it. Saraswati was sweeping me off my feet.

Just so that you can get an idea, let me illustrate various kinds of hypothetical BT-PR patterns in the following diagram. It shows periodic recording of BT and PR. The graph starts out with BT and PR moving in tandem (TP-S).

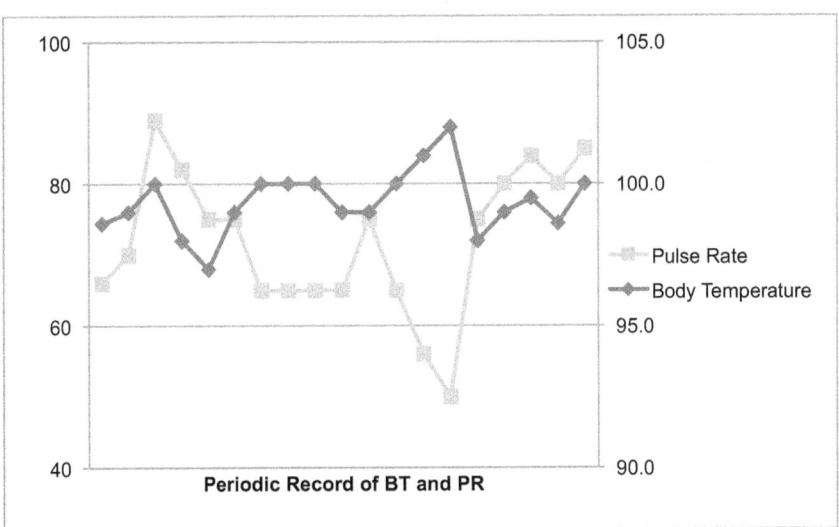

Figure: 1. BT and HR plotted against time are shown. The right vertical axis shows BT in °F and the left one indicates PR. First four intervals show TP-S, Next one is TP-S, one TP-OP, then four TP-Z, and next four show TP-OP with a wide separation of the plots. Last four intervals again show TP-S. TP-OP shows up as a diamond shape, or like reflection of mountains in water, like a mirror image.

---

1   "Mirror-Image relationship between temperature and pulse. JAMA 1979. 242: p. 2760.

TP-S is followed by one TP-OP, then four TP-Z, and next four show TP-OP with a wide separation of the plots. Last four intervals again show TP-S. TP-OP shows up as a diamond shape, or like reflection of mountains in water, like a mirror image. Now on, I may refer to TP-OP as *Diamonds,* and the relationship as *Mirror Image Relationship,* or *MIR.* It is a *reciprocal* or *inverse* relationship.

The reason for the change is, TP-OP looks too scholarly for no good reason and we will be talking about it more often. MIR is the newly observed, nonstandard relationship, unrelated to that occurring in patients with typhoid fever. The latter is only a variant of the conventional relationship.

We did settle the issue whether these diamonds are fake or real. They are real. The next question is, are they of any importance at all, or are just curiosities? Finally, the million dollar question, "Are they girls' or anybody else's best friends, or foes? For answers to these questions, we have to do some more detective work.

6. CUTTING AND POLISHING THE DIAMONDS

Before studying any problem in detail, it is necessary to narrow it down by defining its boundaries and characteristics. We are of course talking about MIR. Graphic records of patients in the ACU display BT and PR recorded every four hours. So there are six time intervals in a day during which we can observe various kinds of BT-PR relationships.

Two out of nine times, MIR can occur by chance alone. For six events, the number is lower. We can consider more than two MIR in a day to be worth looking into. By extending this to one week, we can include the week with four such days with MIR in our review. The inpatients graphs show data for one week at a glance on each page.

Following observations were made:
1. MIR was most likely to appear *after 3-4 days* in patients admitted with fever, pneumonia and systemic infections.
2. Patients with high fever were less likely to show MIR.
3. Those who were described as being dehydrated were less likely to display MIR.
4. In patients with heart failure, or that of kidneys, or liver showed MIR on admission and it became less common with treatment.
5. Patients receiving water pills or *diuretics* were more likely to show MIR, which disappeared when they were given a dose by an injection.
6. Patients on daily weight monitoring for their body water were more likely to show MIR.

7. Just to complete the list, those with MIR were more likely to have a terminal small "s" wave in chest leads #5-6 on their EKGs.

Putting all the above together, it appeared to me that MIR was related to patients' body water in some way. When we are looking at MIR, which is reciprocal or inverse of the conventional relationship, we are looking at the latter, too. In other words, the conventional relationship may also have something to do with body water. That does not lead us anywhere, since BT and PR both are known to be related to body water, more of which can keep the body cooler and less of it can let it over heat.

Water is important for heart to pump the blood. Too much water can increase the load on the heart and slow it down, while too little may make it beat faster to maintain the blood supply to various parts of the body.

Thus, a decrease in body water can accelerate the heart and heat up the body; an increase in water may slow the heart and cool the body. That is the conventional relationship between BT and PR anyway. So, what exactly does the MIR do? Before going further, there is one very important thing a research worker has to learn and that is:

(S)he has to learn to be comfortable with harboring two or more mutually exclusive ideas.

One theory may look correct, to be replaced by another "more correct" one the next day, to come back to the original the day after, is not at all unusual in research. The final selection is only "final" until it is replaced by another. This applies to every step along the entire process and accounts for almost all the fun and torture that research work provides.

Hospital is not a research lab. Its every ward is a chaotic and hectic environment, where patient care is more important than meticulously gathering the academic data. Measurement of water intake, urine output, etc., are not carried out with the precision of a research lab, for understandable reasons.

Graphic record sheets also contain patients' weight, daily water intake and urine output data, charted by the nurses on a daily basis. In sicker patients, intake-output recording is done three times in 24 hours, to coincide with the three shifts of duties of nursing staff.

I have avoided giving any concrete data so far, because as the hypothesis was evolving, data gathering also changed. Tens of records were scrutinized data point by data point to determine the presence or otherwise of the MIR and the frequency of the latter was plotted against intake, output and other variables to see whether there was any connection between them.

If water is important at all, then I figured that atmospheric temperature, relative humidity, etc., may also play a role in BT-PR equation. Along with urine output, the body loses water through visible perspiration, breathing out moist air, in stools and via invisible evaporation from the moist skin. All these are affected by atmospheric factors. Hourly data on these factors are available from the Weather Bureau.

Let us add a few more observations to the list of factors affecting MIR:

1. MIR per eight-hour nursing shift was more common with high water intake in some and with a low one in others.

    This is easy to understand. The conflict arises from the way the body water content is affected by water intake. A patient who is dehydrated can receive lot of water and may still be inadequately hydrated, while another patient who is retaining water can get over-hydrated with a small amount of water intake. In other words, a high water intake can reflect both, over- and under-hydration. Therefore,

2. MIR is probably affected more by body water, or state of hydration, rather than water intake as such.

3. MIR was more likely to occur at lower atmospheric temperature, or on the cooler days. On cooler days, evaporative water loss decreases.

4. MIR is more likely to occur at a higher relative humidity, that is, on muggier days. On such days, the air is nearly saturated with water vapor, unable to absorb more water. That decreases evaporation of water and causes its retention.

    Earlier we had concluded that MIR had something to do with body water. Looking at the above four items, it appears to be related to *increased body water*. Also, we had surmised earlier that the MIR and the conventional relationship both had something to do with body water. Now, if MIR is associated with an excess of body water, then the conventional one may be associated with normal or decreased water. Lest we forget, we still have to talk about the TP-Z in which either BT or PR or both remained unchanged.

The conventional relationship (TP-S) was described by Liebermeister from Germany in 1860s, and is known as *Libermeister's Rule*. Although the rule is quite well known, hardly anyone remembers its discoverer. Let us correct that unacceptable omission right now, by labeling the conventional pattern as LMR (Liebermeister Relationship). So, we have LMR (TP-S) and MIR (TP-OP) two relationships, reciprocal of each other.

Considering the change in BT and in PR over a single interval we had defined TP-OP, TP-S and TP-Z. When many such events take place over several data points, a pattern is established which is described as LMR or MIR. A combination of these two is quite common, but sometimes one or the other grossly predominates.

Combination of *MIR* and *LMR* may occur with very small changes in BT or PR or both. We will refer to that pattern as *"Mixed."* Now on we will use *MIR, LMR* and *"Mixed"* to describe BT-PR patterns and only rarely may use TP-OP, etc., to make a particular point.

LMR exemplifies the Libermeister's rule, and rules generally apply to standard or normal conditions. For example, when talking about water, in physics or chemistry, we talk about the water, one milliliter (ml, or cubic centimeter, cc) of which weighs one gram, boils at 100 °C, and freezes at zero °C. Similarly, Libermeister's rule is expected to be more likely to apply in people with normal hydration.

That leaves the "Mixed" one. What would that reflect? We may be tempted to dismiss that as nothing. In support of TP-Z we should recall that it is the most likely pattern to occur by sheer chance, five out of nine times. Let us look at all three patterns in the real word, as shown in the following figure:

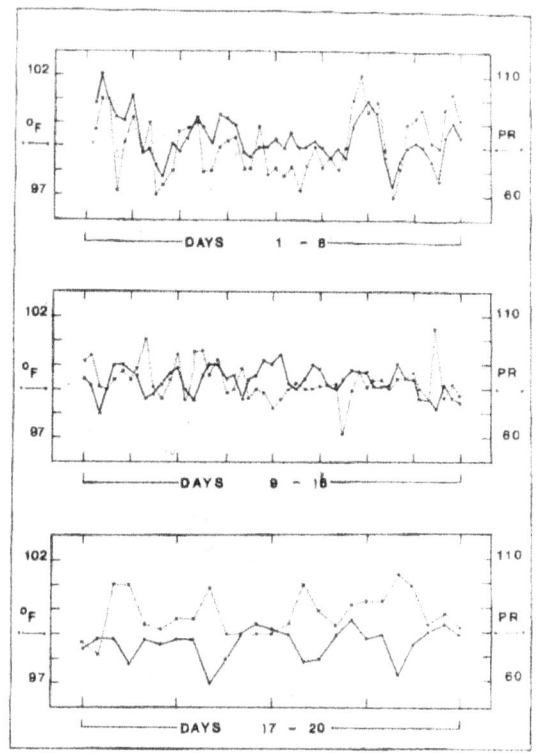

Figure: 2. Temperature pulse record of a patient, redrawn from actual data. The record spans a 20 day period and there are six data points in a day. Solid line indicates BT in °F and the dotted one indicates PR/min. The top panel shows data for days 1-8 and the pattern there is predominantly LMR. The middle panel (days 9-16) shows the "Mixed" pattern with some "diamonds" appearing. The bottom panel (days 17-20) with an expanded scale for the horizontal axis, shows a predominant MIR.

Figure: 2 shows BT-PR record of a patient who was admitted to the ACU with pneumonia, fever, cough and weakness. He was treated with antibiotics and intravenous fluids. He was discharged on the day: 20. Patient's BT is high on admission and it mostly stays around 100 °F. It comes down gradually to go down to 97-98 °F in the bottom panel.

***

If the reader grew up playing with computers, (s)he may not be able to imagine what one had to go through to produce such a diagram for publication. All the lines were drawn in black ink by hand, on a 18 x 24" poster board. The dotted lines representing the PR are from very thin adhesive plastic sheet with broken line printed on it. Strips of required lengths were cut with a one edged blade and manually applied.

Dots to indicate the individual data points were also cut from a thin plastic sheet with rows of dots and circles of different sizes and were applied one by one manually. All letters and numbers are "transfer letters" reverse printed on a thick plastic sheet which was placed on the poster board, letters were properly aligned and then were transferred on to the diagram by applying pressure by rubbing some metallic object over the sheet. Time spent so far, four or five hours.

Even if the art department of the medical college for which I worked had agreed to prepare the diagram for me, it would have charged me $500-600 per diagram at the least. I would have had to pay that from my pockets. Who asked you to do the research without obtaining the grant money?

Next step was to photograph the diagram using a high contrast black and white film, a lights setup to take the photographs, a dark room setup to develop and print the illustrations, everything had to be done by me, including praying that all that would work. Did I mention the expense to set up the dark room? Nowadays, once the data points are entered, the programs like Excel can print this figure out for you in nano seconds. Planning and doing the statistical calculations on my scientific calculator was also my pleasure. Well, rubbing with a hard substance is the only way to make a diamond shine!

7. PROOF OF THE PUDDING

My question to Dr. Ajgaonkar about the typhoid fever was in 1962-63, I started noticing the TP-OP in 1967-68, began studying them in 1972 and now we are entering early 1980s. It took almost a decade to define the hypothesis to be tested, after collecting the data on tens of patients, exploring the role of body water, atmospheric temperature and relative humidity.

Spending days, weeks and months to buy, borrow, or "steal" the necessary equipment, or design it myself with invaluable help from an electrical and electronic engineer, Mr. Sunil Amerasinghe who got an MD degree later to become Dr. Sunil, was quite a fun. Sunil cannibalized an old automatic blood pressure recording machine to enable another old one that could record BT and PR data continually for 72 hours.

He put a clock timer, triggered by a magnetic relay to run the contraption for five minutes every hour to extend the recording period from only six hours to 72 hours. I persuaded him to hide its loose wires attached to a ticking device in its interior, for the fear of emptying out the hospital, even before we got sensitized to the terrorist attacks.

Protecting it from smaller dangers was more difficult. Hospital is a potentially filthy place kept at bay by meticulous and rigorous cleaning. Water pitchers, dinner soup, gravies, coffee mugs, patients' urine and stool, plus lab technicians' blood smudges, all can attack and destroy any record kept for prolonged interval at the patients' bedside.

One morning to our great disbelief and horror, Sunil and I saw our record of the last weekend totally ruined.

There was a carpenter working on something nearby. He had not contributed to the mess. He also shook his head in sympathetic disbelief and asked us why we had not covered it.

We explained that neither of us was a master carpenter and it would have been impossible to get the hospital carpenter shop to do something about it. Next morning we saw a beautifully polished wooden cover with a glass window on top of the recorder.

For recording BT mechanically, Sunil had indicated that if we can insert a thin wire in a thermometer's central channel, it can be connected to an electrical recording system. I visited a thermometer factory in the city, spent the whole day there, discussing various possibilities. A couple of more phone calls to their engineer followed. Then its owner got on the phone to indicate, that was all he could do. He had a business to run, I should have remembered that.

Our automatic device provided the ward nurses with accurate and unbiassed readings of BT and PR, which they seemed to like. However, nurses coming from other hospitals just to do moonlighting and those working on night shifts felt uncomfortable with a strange device that they knew nothing about. Discussions dragged on for a while. Meanwhile, we were able to gather enough data, before removing our contraption.

In a typical mom and pap grocery store fashion, then I studied BT-PR in *healthy normal* (neither of these two terms is welcome in scientific literature which prefers "non-hospitalized" instead) volunteer friends in home setting. Hourly data were collected on BT, PR, fluid intake, urinary output, room temperature and relative humidity. The results were similar to those found in patients.

Since volunteer subjects were not sick in any obvious way, *I concluded that MIR was a physiological phenomenon rather than being a sign of a disease process or a pathological phenomenon.* LMR is known to be physiological to begin with.

After preparing, submitting and resubmitting the research papers to medical journals and accumulating tens of rejection notices, my head was still under water, literally and figuratively and I was having fun, really.

Karl Popper in his "Logic of Scientific Discovery" defines a scientific question as, *a hypothesis presented as a statement which can be disproved.* For example, if the theory states that gravitation pulls everything towards the center of the earth, then a single ball thrown by a child, failing to fall to the ground, effectively disproves it conclusively.

Hypothesis:

We are able to state the hypothesis that *the relationship of body temperature and heart rate is variable, and it can be either LMR, MIR, or "Mixed", depending upon the state of hydration of the individual.* There are several corollaries that follow from this and they can be potentially disproved:

1. LMR and MIR both are physiological processes.
2. Liebermeister's rule does not adequately describe the BT-PR relationship.
3. Relation of BT and PR is a variable one, rather than being fixed.
4. It is affected by state of hydration of the individual.

5. Altering the hydration of an individual is expected to change the pattern of relationship.
6. Overhydration is expected to produce MIR.
7. State of hydration producing LMR and "Mixed" types remains to be seen. One of them is produced by *euhydration* (normal state of hydration). *"Mixed"* or *"Other"* is a more likely candidate (see below) for this.
8. Role of dehydration remains to be seen. LMR's occurring with fever makes it a likely candidate, although being a rule, it is expected to go with the normal state of hydration.

Popper says in his "Logic of Scientific Discovery," that a scientific theory can never be *proved*, but it can always be *disproved*. So, we would try to disprove the validity of the Liebermeister's rule that, *in normal people PR increases with an increase in BT*.

***

We will briefly report here[2] findings and observations on five healthy persons of either sex, studied over three non-consecutive days under various conditions of hydration induced experimentally.

The subjects did not eat or drink anything after dinner the night before. They were weighed on arrival to the hospital lab. A urine sample was collected. Then EKG leads wires were affixed to their chest. EKG monitor displayed the heart rate (HR) continuously. A deep-body thermometer sensor was taped over the chest bone to obtain the body core temperature. Volunteers reclined in hospital bed. They did

---

[2] The full paper appears in part: II.

not eat anything until 5 p.m. when the experiments were concluded.

On one day, they were allowed to drink cool tap water as they pleased (*ad libitum*). On another day, they continued without water until 5 p.m. On third day, after the 8 a.m. and 9 a.m. readings were taken as baseline, they were forced to drink one glass of cool tap water every ten minutes and were encouraged to drink more if they could.

Their water intake, urine output, BT, HR were recorded every half an hour. Urine *osmolality* (salt concentration) was determined using a machine employing the freezing point method. Subjects were weighed again at the end of the experiment.

Five subjects, including three women and two men were studied for total fourteen sessions. One woman had an automobile accident after her second study day, leaving her in continuous pain, leaving the study incomplete. Women were of child bearing age, but not having the menstrual blood flow on the study days. One woman did get her period on the water deprivation day, after the study ended.

No salt or sweetening agents was added to make water more palatable. The latter was allowed to stand for five minutes at room temperature to expel all free air bubbles. When people are asked whether they would like to drink some water, there is a tendency to decline the offer. To avoid that *voluntary dehydration*, subjects were given water in their hands to drink if they wanted to and if the protocol allowed that.

All volunteers were my friends or family members, comfortable with me and they engaged in neutral conversation with me. Water was given in six or eight ounce cups on the day of forced water drinking, depending upon their body weight. One woman did not like to drink water and she threw up, but continued the study regardless.

Records of BT and HR were done on a cue from an automatic timer. Subjects got out of bed to give urine specimen after BT and HR were recorded.

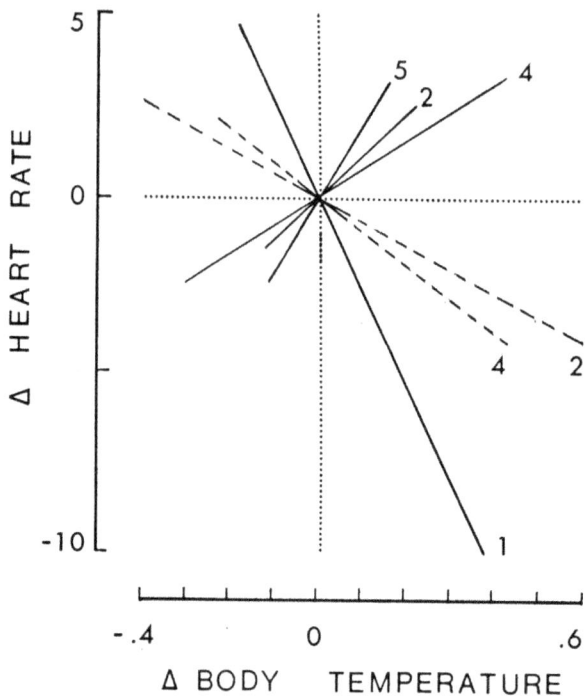

Figure: 3 shows the aggregate data from five subjects, that were statistically significant at p < 0.05. Delta (triangle) refers to "change in" HR or BT during one hour. BT is in °F. Solid lines on the graph show changes in BT and HR when urine osmolality was more than 285 mOsmol/L and the dotted lines show that when osmolality was less than that. Numerals 1-5 refer to subject numbers. Subjects # 2 & 4 showed significant data for high and low osmolality values, while #1 and 5 showed that only for either high or low value of osmolality. Lower right and upper left quadrants are MIR territory and lower left and upper right are the LMR one.

Volunteers # 2 and 4 showed LMR (solid lines) when osmolality was high and MIR (dotted lines) when it was low. Subject # 5 showed LMR with high osmolality. When the body is deprived of water, it conserves the latter by excreting concentrated urine. That is, LMR occurs in presence of a relative lack of water and MIR when there is increased water.

If Liebermeister's rule was valid throughout, practically no data points should have appeared in the upper left and the lower right quadrants. *Presence of statistically significant data in these segments effectively and conclusively disproves the Libermeister's rule.*

***

What about the solid line representing data from the subject # 1? How come that subject's data show an MIR pattern concomitant with high urine osmolality? To make it worse, most of the data points in that subject occurred on the day of water restriction which is expected to cause LMR.

Subject # 1 was a woman who started to have her menstrual period in the evening of the water restriction day. She is also the one who could not tolerate drinking water when she was forced to drink it earlier that day. The way I can explain the aberrant behavior of her data is by invoking *premenstrual retention of water* by her.

What about her high urine osmolality which indicates low body water? It seems to me that the way the body retains water in the premenstrual period is by excreting less of it, thereby making the urine more concentrated. In her case, high osmolality indicates an attempt at retaining water, successful one at that. Water restriction for a few hours that day by me was apparently not enough to correct her retained water and hence the MIR. This point itself requires further study.

We have shown that BT-HR relationship is affected probably not by urinary osmolality as such, but by body water indicated by it. Our data do not deal with body water directly.

***

The question comes up, "What is the normal relation between BT and HR, when body water, as indicated by urinary osmolality, is normal (280 msmol/L)? Neither LMR nor MIR can represent that, since they both are related to decreased and increased body water respectively.

Well, still there is one more candidate to make that claim and that is TP-Z in which either BT or HR or both may remain unchanged. Where would TP-Z be in figure: 3? On the fence, seriously, between MIR and LMR, that is, on the vertical and horizontal axes! The vertical axis represents the zero value of $\triangle$BT while the horizontal one that of $\triangle$HR. The point of origin, where the axes intersect is the point where the value of $\triangle$BT and $\triangle$HR both is zero.

All this adds up to show that *there is no relation between BT and HR as such.* Normally, the pattern toggles between MIR and LMR, with neither of them dominating. With sustained overhydration or underhydration, MIR or LMR gets established. BT-HR or BT-PR relationship is a perfectly balanced "seesaw" between LMR and MIR respectively.

***

It is incumbent upon the one who disproves a theory, to explain how the supposedly wrong theory came into being and how it could get accepted. In Libermeister's time

44

during mid 1860s, infections were rampant, there were no antibiotics or intravenous fluids. High fevers were common.

Moreover, many fevers were treated by withholding oral intake. As if that was not enough, blood letting and purging were applied therapeutically. Fevers themselves could make patients lose water. Diarrhea associated with many infections would worsen the dehydration, associated vomiting would aggravate that still further and prevent oral hydration. There were enough reasons for dehydration to occur and none to ameliorate it.

Most if not all of Liebermeister's patients—they were certainly not normal people—were dehydrated in varying severity. When he chose patients with fevers, he was inadvertently selecting dehydrated individuals. In our patients and healthy volunteers, we did confirm the occurrence of LMR in presence of decreased body water.

As noted earlier, MIR was less commonly seen with fevers. Anecdotally, I did see a couple of times patients with fevers receiving intravenous fluids, display MIR, probably attributable to excess body water.

***

How can we explain the relative bradycardia (slow heart) associated with the typhoid fever? To recall, it is an LMR pattern, but the rise in PR is less than what is expected. That is, there is a tendency of the pattern to shift towards MIR, albeit unsuccessfully. The lack of success may be due to high fever, vomiting and poor intake keeping the volume of body water relatively low. The relatively slow heart may be caused by say, fluid retention taking place in case of typhoid fever. This needs to be confirmed or otherwise, but it is likely.

The word "typhoid" means "like typhus (a cloud)" referring to the patient's mental status, probably caused by water logging of the brain. Typhoid fever is characterized by gastrointestinal symptoms also and there are several receptors in abdomen to affect the water balance. Antidiuretic hormone (ADH) which promotes water retention, may be playing a part.

Viral hepatitis and Legionnaire's disease both of which are associated with an abdominal illness, are also known to produce relative bradycardia. Our data do not allow us to comment beyond a conjecture. It is hoped that future research workers may want,

1. To investigate LMR and MIR as affected by the body water, with modern equipment and tests to confirm or refute the findings presented here.
2. To see whether typhoid and other conditions just mentioned are associated with water retention and whether correcting that, if deemed appropriate, produces LMR.
3. To explore whether LMR or MIR is more common in patients with hypothermia, induced or otherwise, as opposed to with fever. I would postulate, it will be MIR, based on what we have just seen.
4. The 'diamonds" may indicate presence of overhydration in patients. This should be confirmed or ruled out by standard tests.
5. To generate other ideas from this and to investigate them, and to learn not to ignore the basic science, no matter how sophisticated the medicine gets.

8. ELECTROCARDIOGRAM (EKG)
MAKING AND BREAKING WAVES WITH WATER

There has been lot of talk about importance of motivation, determination and perseverance or the "stick-to-itiveness." Among the volunteers who came for the BT-HR study, there was a woman social worker who was working on the same ward as I did. She did not drive to work and was dropped off by her father. She lived 15 miles from the hospital. The research work was done on the weekends, for which none of us got any pay, leave aside the overtime.

I offered to pick her up from her house which was in an entirely different direction, on that Saturday but she firmly declined. I started my car from my home and drove for maybe a mile, with 18 more miles to go, when suddenly, its engine quit. In those days before the arrival of the cell-phone, there was no way for me to contact her. If she reached the hospital, she had no way to get into the part of the hospital where the deserted lab was located.

For a few minutes, I just waited, worried about the wasted weekend, without producing anything and afraid that she may refuse to come again. I looked at the steering wheel as if to plead my case. Although it had no control over the engine, it did hold the ignition key. The car did not start in response to my several attempts and I was worried about running down the battery.

I knew there was only one way out. The car had to start. I grabbed the steering wheel in desperation, held it very tightly and shook it violently, warning at the same time, "You better start, right now! I have no time to pamper you. If you don't start now, I am going to leave you right here!" and pinched the key twisting it simultaneously. The car started! It got the message and must have realized that I meant business. I made it in due time.

***

Much has been said about the role of chance, accident or serendipity in research, medical and other. A consensus has emerged that these do play a significant role, provided they occur to a prepared mind, creative enough to connect the dots and appreciate the relevance of a chance observation.

Before asking the volunteers to drink a large amount of water forcibly, it was necessary to determine how much water a person could tolerate. My neighbor and friend Dr. Gurunanjappa Bale, whom we called *Guru* for short, came with me on one weekend to help me out. We had to do a dry run of the experiment.

He was going to give me water, etc. I was to try to drink as much water as I could. Cardiac monitor leads were applied to my chest and I reclined on the hospital bed. The monitor was behind and above my head, not easily visible to me. We were using the monitor only to read off the heart rate from it rather than taking the pulse each time.

Guru was an actuarial statistician working for a major life insurance company and he knew more about the mortality data than vital signs of a living person. He kept on giving me water and I kept on drinking it. He stared at me in disbelief, since he already had had a hard time drinking much water the previous weekend.

He was aware of the discussion we had about a potential volunteer who had low thyroid function (*hypothyroidism*) and we were debating whether it would be safe to force water on her. He had no idea how to tell whether I was getting into trouble thanks to drinking all that water. Therefore, he kept on looking at the monitor without quite knowing what to expect.

After I drank a few more glasses, he looked at the monitor, with a wrinkled forehead and squinted eyes and told me, "I don't know Dr. Shah, what to make of this, but these monitor waves look much smaller since you drank so much water!"

"Well, you are the one who saw the change. I am feeling fine. The only thing we can do is to check again at the end of the experiment to see whether the amplitude regains its original height." I instructed him. He did confirm later in the day without any hesitation that his observation was indeed valid.

Cardiac monitors are capable of doing all kinds of things, including erroneously displaying a straight line, thereby indicating the patient's death, "rather prematurely and with great deal of exaggeration."

Monitors are looked at to check the heart rhythm and rate, and nothing more. Change in the amplitude of its waves is better appreciated on the regular printed EKG. The change was probably not small. It is not easy for someone unfamiliar with looking at the monitor, to notice the change in the size of the waves, from a distance of ten feet—he was near the foot and the monitor was near the head end of the bed—and to muster the courage to point it out to a doctor, at the same time fearing getting an evasive sleigh of my hand to indicate, "Oh, that is nothing!"

I do not mean to claim that I am different or better than others, but any doctor would have done just that, although there is no justification or basis to do so, at least, not in a research lab, anyway. When I instructed Guru to look at it again when I was done excreting all that water, to see whether the waves got larger again, I had a valid reason to believe him.

A few days earlier, I had read an article in a medical journal, describing a new method to assess the volume of the body water in the kidney dialysis patients. The method consisted of introducing a miniscule amount of electric current at one point on the body and picking it up at another to see how much of it was lost because of the body's resistance to electricity. This is known as *bioimpedence* which could indirectly tell one the amount of body water. Instead of the introduced current, what Guru saw was the drop in voltage of body's own electric current. It made sense.

The reason I had read that esoteric paper was, I was working on modifying the peritoneal dialysis to remove carbon dioxide from patients with respiratory failure (we will get to it a few chapters later) and I was doing the preliminary work on influence of body water on BT-HR relationship. I was at the confluence of water, kidneys, and heart. So much for the role of accidents and chance in research.

***

On the following Monday, I revised the experimental protocol and requested the Research Committee to allow me to do EKG every hour on the volunteers, which was approved immediately. Water is a very good insulator and its accumulation around the heart and the lungs is known to cause a low voltage in the EKG.

It would be good and easy to report this insulating effect of body water in the same or another paper, I thought.

Just as I had naively thought of writing up MIR as an insignificant chance event! Saraswati was at it, again.

Hourly EKGs were added to the protocol of the BT-PR study. They were done after recording BT and PR and before the subject got up to pass urine. The EKG tracing of each heart beat consists of mainly five waves called P-Q-R-S-T. The P wave reflects activity of the receiving chambers, *atria* of the heart and the QRS (written as, qRs) represents that of the ejecting chambers, called *ventricles*. The T-wave represents the electrical recovery of the latter.

There are 12 EKG leads, all of which were recorded for 8-10 beats hourly for 10 times during the test day. Amplitude or the height of each wave was measured in a standardized fashion and plotted on a graph against urinary osmolality, a proxy for body water. *Almost all leads in all volunteers showed significant correlations with body water on the regression analysis.*

That should have been the end of it. However, there was one problem. With increased body water, some waves got bigger, rather than getting smaller thanks to the insulating effect of water as expected. Now your hand is stuck in the cookie jar!

Let me show you a few illustrations of changes in the amplitude that were visible on simple inspection, unlike the minute changes mentioned above. *Such changes, as shown in figures 4-7, were not common* in healthy volunteers studied.

In figure: 4, the sharp wave going slightly up and then down is the qRs complex. A very small wave just before (to our left) that and rising just above the baseline is the P wave and the curvy peak behind (to our right) the qRs, is the T wave.

All figures show the resting EKG at the top, the middle panel shows the EKG when subject had taken maximal amount of water and the bottom panel shows the EKG after the excess water was voided.

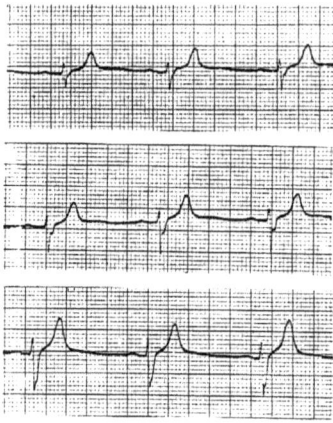

Figure: 4. Note that the qRs complex gets progressively larger from the top to the bottom panel. It is known to show this daily rhythm. This is probably unrelated to water drinking. QRS also grows through all panels. The P wave appears to remain unchanged.

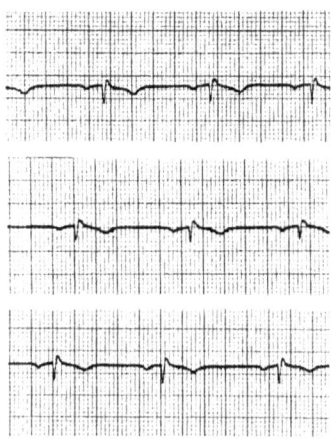

Figure: 5. Notice that the qRs dipping downwards gets smaller in the middle panel and is restored in the lowest one. The upswing also changes, but that may be difficult to appreciate.

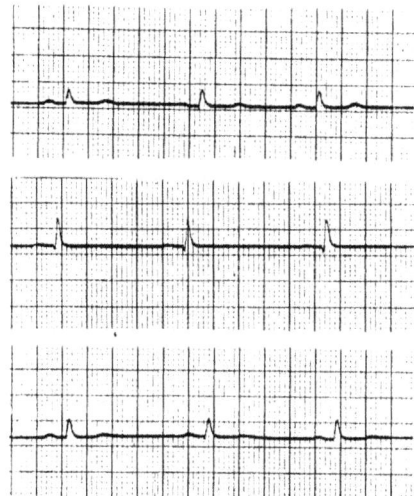

Figure: 6. The QRS amplitude increases with forced water intake (middle panel) and returns to the baseline value in the bottom panel. Also note that the P wave preceding the QRS disappears in the middle panel, to return in the bottom one. The same is the case with the T wave which follows the QRS. The T wave begins to reappear in the bottom panel.

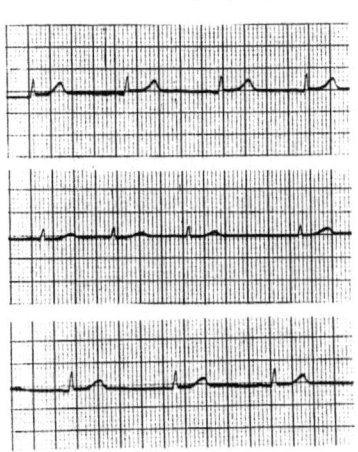

Figure: 7. The QRS gets smaller, its earlier part dipping down in the top panel disappears in the middle one and reappears in the bottom panel. The QRS itself gets smaller and then returns to normal, from top to bottom. The domed T wave after the QRS gets flattened in the middle panel and then comes back to its original shape in the bottom panel.

The problem was getting more fascinating. When Einthovan (pronounced as *Einhoffen*) invented the EKG, he knew that the EKG recorded off the skin was not the same as the one recorded off the heart directly. For making it practical, he had to assume that the chest is a uniform or *homogeneous* structure, that is, heart, lungs, muscle, blood, all are equal conductors of electricity.

Not that he did not know the truth, but such assumptions are always being made just for the argument. When we say the men and women are same, we know quite well that they are not. The heart muscle is ten times better conductor than the lungs full of air and blood in the heart chambers is four times better conductor than the heart muscle. This variations or *heterogenicity* of organs modify the electric waves on their way to the body surface.

As we tend to walk on the neatly trimmed lawn as a short cut rather than walking on the designated paths, electric current likes to do that, too. Rather than going along the heart muscle, it jumps through the blood in the cavity, thereby making the wave form smaller. Similarly, the current flowing across the wall of the heart muscle is amplified. This is known as *Brody's Effect*. I learned that subsequently while reviewing the literature.

Brody's effect can explain why some waves got bigger, while others got smaller. What has body water to do with this? Water changes the concentration of blood in the cavity. Although commonly known to be an insulator, water is many fold better conductor than the red blood cells.

***

What is the significance of these findings? I came across a case report[3] of a very sick patient who needed to have blood transfusion. In patients with weak heart, it may be dangerous to transfuse blood, because that may over burden the heart, which in turn may fail. Patient's EKG did show that patient's left ventricle, the main pumping chamber was indeed strained.

The bag of blood was already on the ward, when the chief resident on his way home got the EKG report. He told the senior night doctor about it, suggesting to withhold the transfusion. Before the message could trickle down to the intern, the latter transfused the blood.

Fortunately, nothing untoward happened and the patient got better. Next day, the chief resident was aghast to hear the entire story. He ordered an EKG to be done right away, called *Stat*. The left ventricular strain pattern had disappeared. An EKG finding based on the voltage of the waves had misled doctors to withhold a life saving intervention!

Doctors use voltage criteria to diagnose over burdened ventricles. Such chambers become very thick before failing completely. This thickening is known as *hypertrophy* and it shows up on EKG as increased amplitude or voltage in certain leads. It is known that these voltage criteria are not very reliable.

EKG tracings show many day-to-day variations and even beat-by-beat variations that are poorly understood. There are reports in the literature of a missed beat being followed by a qRs of greater magnitude. Many such variations may be due to changes in the volume of blood within the

---

[3] I have been unable to find this report again among my filing cabinets or in the literature search.

heart or those in its conductivity caused by *anemia,* which dilutes it.

In my sojourn as a physician in the long term care Coler Hospital, I had seen many old patients with pneumonia or other infection and fever being admitted under my care, with very high amplitude of EKG waves in the chest leads[4]. After they were treated with antibiotics and intravenous fluids to hydrate them, the EKG amplitude came down to their pre-illness size.

To avoid the effect of food and fluid, most blood tests are done on fasting blood specimen. Maybe the EKG should be done during the fasting or otherwise standardized condition to improve its reliability.

What are the implications of the data and findings presented here? Let us enumerate:

1. We have conclusively shown that amplitude of various EKG waves is affected by body water.
2. These water related changes in amplitude may explain some, if not all, day-to-day variations in EKG.
3. Some beat-to-beat variations have been shown to have been caused by change in volume of blood within the heart.
4. Voltage criteria to diagnose left ventricular hypertrophy, right ventricular strain, etc., are not reliable, partly because the amplitude is so variable.

---

[4] There are three electrodes placed, one on each shoulder and on the left leg, which individually and then in three pairs constitute six leads. The other six are almost all placed on the left front chest wall and are called the *chest leads.*

5. An EKG taken under standard condition of hydration may be more dependable, at least in some selected cases.

6. Basic science implications of these findings need to be assessed further.

These findings regarding body water and its influence on BT-PR relationship and on EKG amplitude were published as abstracts in the Clinical Research[5]. A letter to the editor of the Journal of the AMA (JAMA) reporting on MIR not being a chance event was also published, as mentioned before. Full papers sent to several journals were rejected, and are included in part: II.

---

5   Changes in the amplitude of electrocardiographic waves induced by forced water intake
     Clinical Research. 1986. 34:343A.

     Variability of body temperature — heart rate relationship induced by changes in the water balance.
     Clinical Research. 1986. 34:343A.

9. RESPIRATION
THE MOST IMPORTANT VITAL SIGN

Vital signs include temperature, pulse and respiration, *TPR* in short. We have gone over the new findings, observations and results of experimental data on effect of body water on BT-PR relationship and on amplitude of the waves on the EKG.

The body is kept warm by tissues metabolizing the food we eat. That heat is carried throughout the body by pumping action of the heart. For producing heat by burning fuel first we need oxygen and for that we have to breathe. They do not talk about "breath of life" for nothing.

The blueprint of our lives are prepared very early in our lives, unbeknownst to us. You don't have to believe in destiny, but there is something that makes sure that, "Events cast their shadows first." My asking about typhoid fever was one such event.

Another such event had taken place a few months before that at the end of the first MBBS. Our professor of physiology, Dr. T. H. Rindani, one of the best teachers I ever had, gave us an assignment for our summer vacation to write a long thesis on the topic of our choice. That was to be my first long paper in medicine. I chose "Pulmonary Vascular Bed and Circulation," or blood vessels of the lungs.

In comparison to the systemic one, the pulmonary circulation receives scant little attention in physiology lectures. The systemic circulation providing blood to our brain, kidneys, liver, stomach, sense organs and even to the heart itself is a huge system of giant blood vessels like the aorta and it works at very high pressure—commonly known as *blood pressure*, the famous 120/80 one. It carries oxygen and food material all over the body. Its veins bring the waste products and carbon dioxide back to the heart.

The same amount of blood, five liters every minute, now goes to the right side of the heart, to be pumped through large sponge like lungs mostly full of air, at one-tenth the pressure and then return to the heart. Lungs must be very important to receive such enormous blood flow.

The systemic arteries carry oxygenated, bright red blood and veins carry the blue blood with far less oxygen. However, the pulmonary *veins* carry bright red blood to the heart and the pulmonary *artery* is the only one in the body to carry the blue blood. Ancient people knew this quite well, albeit without appreciating its significance clearly.

The word *artery* implies the "one that carries air," or oxygen. The systemic arteries do that, pulmonary artery does not. They used to call pulmonary artery as the *venous artery* and the veins as the *arterial veins*. It is a fascinating system. The heart itself receives its own blood supply through the coronary arteries after it is done pumping the blood to the rest of the body, like a good wife or mother eating only after feeding her family.

I filled my paper with fascinating details gathered from the papers written by the "Who is who" in pulmonary physiology and medicine, without realizing it then. I pre-pared an artistic cover page (figure on the next page), that I was going to keep dearly to date.

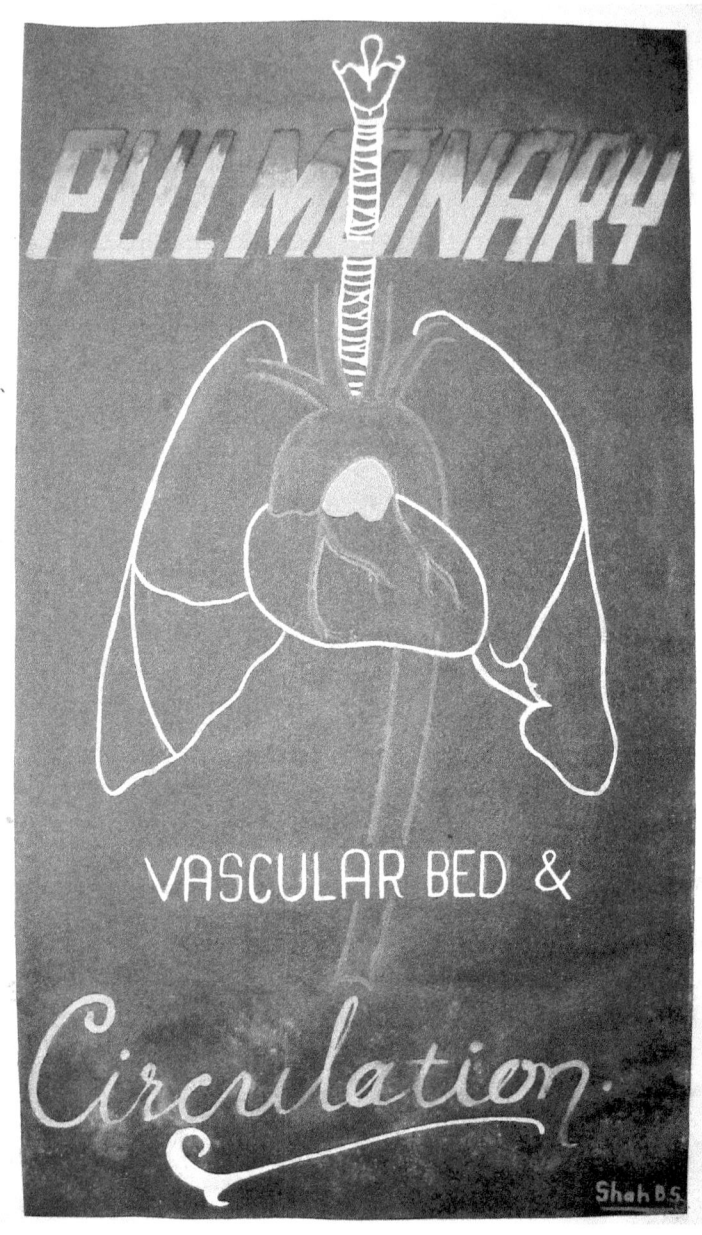

I do not quite remember when I first learned about the similarity[6] between hemoglobin in our blood and chlorophyl in the plant world. Both are made of four pentagons with their peaks meeting at one point. For these pentagons, you have to visualize the way children draw a house—a square, with a triangular roof over it.

Where the four such houses drawn on a paper meet, there is an iron molecule (Fe) in case of *heme* of our hemoglobin, globin being a protein. Replace the iron molecule with magnesium (Mg) and you get chlorophyl. Mother nature, or some other creator made the plant and the animal kingdoms with just a sleigh of the hand!

Plants with chlorophyl take up carbon dioxide and give out oxygen for us. "In the beginning" there was only carbon dioxide produced from volcanic eruptions. Plants produced oxygen from it for us. We return the favor by producing carbon dioxide again. Isn't all this extremely marvelous! To me, it has always been. This page is the complete ecology and environmental sciences in brief.

***

During my second year medical residency training in what was New York Infirmary in lower Manhattan, we used to rotate through the Manhattan V. A. Hospital a mile up north, for three months to be exposed to the pulmonary medicine. Besides learning my favorite subject, I liked the people there and signed up for a two year fellowship.

While in the med school, I was also fascinated by the acid-base physiology and the buffer system. Carbon dioxide

---

6   I believe that happened a decade or more after I became a doctor. The exact circumstances of the revelation escape me now, but I do remember that moment quite vividly.

is also known as "carbonic *acid* gas." It is the gas in colas and sodas we drink. It is acidic. Our tissues produce lot of carbon dioxide which the venous blood has to carry to the heart.

Do you ever wonder, why there is so much fizz in the soda bottle? Why does the liquid rush out together with gas on opening the can, especially after shaking it a bit? The gas is under high pressure, which is suddenly released on opening the cap. The sparkling taste is due to the compressed carbon dioxide which is poorly soluble in water, but its solubility increases directly in line with applied pressure.

By the time blood reaches the veins, almost all pressure of the blood is gone. We would need maybe ten times our blood volume to carry all that gas in solution. Moreover, that solution would be too acidic. Mother nature likes to keep our internal environment, *mileu interiore* bathing our tissues to be relatively unchanged at temperature 98.6 °F and acidity level at pH 7.40.

Body converts the acidic carbon dioxide into a less acidic and far more soluble bicarbonate. You may recall from your high school chemistry that carbonates are alkaline, but bicarbonates are less so (*bi-* means acid, bicarbonate is *acidic alkali*). Then this less acidic blood is carried by veins to the heart and then to the lungs where the process is reversed and carbon dioxide is given up.

Most of us had found this fascinating chapter very confusing, partly because we had no facility to measure the arterial blood gases, or the ABGs in Mumbai then. It was very common in the U.S.A. to do the ABGs on a blood sample drawn from an artery, as opposed to the usual blood work drawn from a vein. We did ABGs very frequently on our sick patients in the ICU and on the respiratory wards in the U.S.

Once I had a critically ill respiratory patient with severe emphysema. He was getting worse and was in need of a respirator. I drew a blood sample, but the procedure turned out to be more difficult than what I had expected it to be. The syringe had a bad lock. I managed to take the sample to the lab, where our lab technician Linda (short for Olinda) ran the tests. The result was unbelievable. The blood sample showed nearly normal level of gases, in a moribund patient!

I shook my head in disbelief. Linda asked me to draw another specimen, which I did and it showed the level of gases to be as bad as they could be. That was not a rare event, as both of us knew so well. Room air leaking into a sample vitiates the results. Still, I was greatly disturbed from then on and kept talking about it. My senior physicians advised me not to take it to my heart, since it was not a major error and that I had done everything right.

No. There was indeed, something wrong, grossly wrong. This was a patient in the ICU, with respiratory failure that was about to kill him, one whom we were planning to put on a respirator through a tracheostomy tube in his neck, taking away his ability to talk.

Why all that? Just to normalize oxygen and carbon dioxide levels in his blood, with little hope for a lasting success. On the other hand, exposing that blood accidently to a small bubble of air was enough to make his blood gases nearly normal. What could be simpler and easier than that!

Many ideas in medicine have come out of doctor's unbearable frustration coming from helplessly caring for their dying patients and wondering, "Isn't there anything,

anything at all that I can do to help these patients?" The answer does not come right away. The question refuses to go away, until one day, the doctor himself or herself almost becomes the answer.

The question begins to assume a definite concrete form like, "Only if we can join the aorta and *vena cava* (the main vein) near the heart," or "I wish there was a way to stop the heart during the surgery." In the case of our patient, it was, *Why can't we expose the patient's blood to the air?*

I did not see any problem with doing just that. In my medical college hospital, I had seen blood being transfused from an open funnel into patient's body. In the U.S. I had seen the blood dripping through a small cylindrical chamber in the intravenous tubing. There was no reason why we could not run air through that or another similar device.

The idea of leaving the blood exposed to air for long was not appealing to me. Infection, clotting, cooling, etc., may pose problems. I liked to mimic mother nature by keeping the air and blood separated by a thin membrane.

There was a renal dialysis unit in the V. A. Hospital. I met its technical chief to pick his brain. I asked about using air instead of saline solution in the outer tank. He said that it could be done, but he wondered what I was trying to do. I explained it to him. He said, "You can use the oxygenators." I had heard about them, although very few doctors then were really aware of them as practical devices. I did not know whether they were available in the market.

They were not. Only a few research labs working under contracts with the government or the industry had access to them, while I was working on my own with no real money. Finally, I learned that Edwards Lab in California was marketing two animal models of the Lande´-Edwards membrane lung. They came in one or three square meter membrane size.

This may sound very familiar today, but it was then a frighteningly uncharted territory even for the experts in the field. I had to do animal experiments on dogs to develop the system. I could not even kill a mouse, roach, or even an ant with impunity. I was born and brought up in a staunch vegetarian Jain[7] family, but I had learned to do what I had to do, leaving my personal beliefs in abeyance. I was not doing this for money, fame, or something like that. I was going to do something that only I could do, then.

Research committee approved the project and some seed money for buying the necessary equipment and dogs. A woman attending physician was going to work as my senior researcher. I do not know which one of us hated it more to see a dog die. It was very painful. There was no possibility of using the same animal repeatedly. The animal behavior and our facilities would not allow that.

Oxygenators were used in the open heart surgery to maintain the oxygenation of blood, taking over the function of the patient's own lungs. Membrane oxygenators were found to be less damaging to blood, as compared to the open air, or the bubble type. Bubble type machines blew away carbon dioxide and created problems, while the membrane units were limited in their removal of carbon dioxide.

Decades later, the process of oxygenation was going to be known as Extracorporeal Membrane Oxygenation (ECMO, pronounced as *Ekmo*). It is a highly complex proce-

---

[7]   See "An Introduction to Jainism" in the end pages.

dure, requiring removing the entire cardiac output about five liters of blood every minute from the body, pump it through various devices and after treating it with 100% oxygen, returning it to patient's cannulated major blood vessels, making sure the blood does not clot.

Hypothesis:

My idea was different and the hypothesis went along these lines of reasoning.

1. Oxygenation is not the primary purpose, but removal of carbon dioxide is the aim.

2. Bubble oxygenators would be better for that purpose, however, membrane lungs were easy on the blood and may be better suited for eventual long term use to provide respiratory support in patients with ventilator (respirator) to wean patients off that.

3. We should be able to work with much lower blood flow rate.

4. We should be able to use the room air, instead of oxygen with its severe complications.

5. In the anesthetized animals whose respiration was experimentally curtailed to produce low oxygen level and high carbon dioxide level, when we lower the carbon dioxide level using membrane oxygenators, such animals' oxygen level should automatically improve.

6. Eventually it should be possible to make a portable device to restore freedom of speech and mobility to respiratory patients.

It was incumbent upon me to digest a very complex physiological process, master a highly technical cutting-edge process, and modify the latter to make it work. To recall, I had practically never seen a heart-lung bypass in any detail. Again, only the basic science was guiding me along.

There is a big fundamental difference between giving oxygen to and removing carbon dioxide from the blood. Giving oxygen is comparable to feeding people. If you have to feed 100 people, you cannot overstuff one and tell him to share it with the rest.

Removing carbon dioxide, on the other hand, is like collecting money. If you want to collect one dollar from each of the 100 people, you can take all of $100 from one person who can then collect one dollar from each one.

That means, if we want to remove carbon dioxide, we can deal with very little blood flow. Our body at rest produces about 200 ml of carbon dioxide every minute. About 100 ml of blood contains nearly 50 ml of it. Therefore, theoretically we can remove 200 ml of carbon dioxide from only 400 ml or two glassfuls of blood, instead of the entire cardiac output of more than ten times as much.

In a patient who is still breathing on his own, we may not need to remove all 200 ml of carbon dioxide either, only a fraction of that may suffice. This amount was labeled by me as *Ventilatory Deficit*.

Let me give a practical example here. Say, someone makes $500 a week, and has to spend $550. He works extra hours to make $50. However, he has to spend more on gasoline to go to that other job, and has to buy extra coffee, and has to pay extra income tax, leaving him with only $30 additional. He can do yet one more job to earn $30 more to have $20 in his hands.

His problem is not $500, nor is it $550, nor $580. His problem is only $50. If someone could give him $50 every week (or if he can decrease his weekly expenses by that much), he would live happily ever after. This figure, $50 is his *financial deficit*. The *ventilatory deficit* is also something like that.

When lungs cannot remove carbon dioxide adequately, its level in the alveoli and then in the blood rises. That increases the transfer of the gas to establish the balance. When you remove the amount of gas responsible for raising its level, the level normalizes. This is the practical meaning of *ventilatory deficit*.

Gas transfer across a membrane depends on its *gradient* or difference in the relative concentration on either side of the membrane. Since 100% oxygen or the room air neither of which contain any carbon dioxide, either of them can provide the same gradient for removal of carbon dioxide and allow us to use the room air on the gas phase.

10. HEMORESPIRATORS

The artificial lung used for giving oxygen is called an *oxygenator*. I was going to use it for removal of carbon dioxide. Both these functions collectively are known as respiration and since blood was going to be used directly, I coined the term *Hemo (blood) Respirator*. Ventilation is movement of air. Removal of carbon dioxide depends upon that. Therefore respirators used for emphysema patients are called *Ventilators*, rather than respirators.

I wish I can share with you the excitement of planning and designing an experimental project single handedly, getting it approved while still being in training and later on executing it successfully. We have now returned to 1971-72, ten years before the BT-PR-EKG experiments. The Pulmonary Service at the V.A. Hospital provided me with a cart to carry the gas cylinders, the blood gas analyzer, many tubes, wires and other gadgets.

The research lab assistant was a pro in handling the animals, anesthetizing them and inserting breathing tubes in their airways. My senior researcher was highly skilled and experienced in running the experiments. I had learned handling of gases from the Respiratory Therapy department and had borrowed and learned to use the highly precise blood gas analyzer from the lab and had acquired a rudimentary knowledge of replacing its expensive and balky electrodes and doing minor troubleshooting as well.

First couple of experiments were for creating and perfecting the experimental circuit. Under high pressure from the pumps, the tubing often gave way showering me with not so holy water initially and giving me a blood bath later on. At times there were floor to ceiling blood splashes, something that I had never seen, nor had expected to see. Membrane lungs also ruptured under high pressures applied inadvertently. Eventually, with my increasing knowledge about fluid pressures, hydrodynamics, pressure gradients and so on, things began to work.

Original plan was to curtail the respiration of the dogs to raise their carbon dioxide. That worked, but the animal died before we could even start the circuit. Then we decided to start the circuit first and then reduce the ventilation to 50% or less as tolerated and attempted to balance that by removing carbon dioxide. On discontinuing the circuit, animals died of very high carbon dioxide level, indicating what the procedure was keeping it at bay.

There was nothing new in membrane lungs giving respiratory support. What was new was the very low blood flow rate (50-300 ml/min) used, which was totally inadequate for achieving oxygenation. Also, we were able to use compressed air on the gas phase without any difficulty in removing carbon dioxide.

My senior researcher was never able to get into it. She confessed she did not have the slightest idea what I was up to, but then admitted that I apparently did. Even after several attempts, I could not communicate with her and even after the experiments worked, she had trouble appreciating their significance. She did help me through the entire project though.

Several experiments were side tracked at her insistence for determining and calculating the variables like cardiac output, which were of no use, nor were they in the protocol. The Research Committee refused to renew the project, which I believed was on the right track and was near its successful conclusion. I presented my case respectfully and candidly to the Chief of the Pulmonary Service, who in turn personally went to the Committee and got the project extended.

Meanwhile I had moved to The Coler Memorial Hospital. My Chief there, Dr. Lothar Wertheimer was very supportive and he allowed me to go to the V. A. Hospital one day a week. That was not popular with the administration, understandably. I did manage to complete the project.

As was the tradition going to be, I manually prepared and photographed the illustrations myself. A paper reporting the findings was prepared and sent to several journals from 1972 to 1985. There were very few journals that published this kind of papers, especially from a novice. Most of the published papers dealt with oxygenation rather than with removal of carbon dioxide primarily.

The American Society for Artificial Internal Organs (ASAIO) published abstracts of papers only from its members or those sponsored by its members. Becoming its member was not an option, because you have to had published at least two papers related to the artificial organs.

My senior researcher had the same problem with the manuscript as she did with the experiments. After several futile discussions and endless delay in reaching any resolution, I finally suggested that I should continue to work on the manuscript, submit it for publication and if, and when it is accepted, then I would contact her about adding her name as a co-author. When it was, she declined, giving me the full credit. I am deeply indebted for her support, and am saddened at not being able to have her as my co-author.

Finally an abstract of Hemorespirators[8] was published in the Transactions of the ASAIO, sponsored by Dr. Arnold Lande´, the inventor of the membrane lung that I had used. The full paper was published[9] in the last issue of the prestigious journal of ASAIO, in December, 1985.

There was a reason why that journal was closing down. The National Library of Medicine which produces the Index Medicus, the massive 25 volume database of articles published in all 50-60,000 medical journals from around the world, included only the *peer reviewed* journals, that is, the expert peers in the field had critically evaluated those papers.

The papers published by the ASAIO Journal were reviewed by the peers, but not in a way that was satisfactory to the indexing authorities. A new journal was going to and did replace the old one.

For me, the paper that was published after waiting for almost 15 years, in the most prestigious journal of the best known organization in the field of the artificial organs, was not going to show up in any search of the literature. Even nearly 25 plus years after it was "published," one still may not be able to find it.

Even though the paper is not easily available, I am not at liberty to present here the details of results of the experi-

---

8   Correction of experimental hypercapnia and hypoxemia with membrane lung
      ASAIO Abstracts. 1985. 14; p. 67.

9   A simplified extracorporeal approach to experimental ventilatory failure.
      ASAIO Journal. 1985; 223-227.

ments, since they constitute copyrighted material of the ASAIO Journal that does not exist at present.

Let us review what was achieved by those experiments:

1. Hemorespirators can be effectively used primarily to remove carbon dioxide.
2. High blood flow rates and high concentration of oxygen necessary for achieving oxygenation, making the procedure highly complex, are not necessary for Hemorespirators.
3. For carbon dioxide removal, compressed air and 50-300 ml/min flow of blood would suffice.
4. On correcting the high level of carbon dioxide in blood produced by acute hypoventilation, the oxygen level also gets corrected.
5. Oxygenation thus achieved cannot be credited to the Hemorespirator, since the conditions were not conducive for that. That oxygen was transfered by animals' own lungs.
6. To correct the retention of carbon dioxide induced by *hypoventilation* of animals, it is not necessary to extract the total production of carbon dioxide every minute (200 ml). Extracting a small fraction of it, the *ventilatory deficit* is sufficient.
7. Extracorporeal circulation was brought out of the cardiothoracic operating room to the renal dialysis level, which can be handled by a trained physician.

11. KISSING "GOOD BYE" TO BLOOD

Even though the hemorespirators did simplify the extracorporeal removal of carbon dioxide to bring it within the reach of physicians, it still required handling the blood. Dialysis physicians have been doing it for decades now, but our experiments took place in the early 1970s. Dialysis for kidney failure is a life sustaining procedure that can also be used as a *bridger technology* to renal transplant and a fallback option should the transplant fail for some reason.

The driving force behind the Hemorespirators was, to do for the failure of the lungs what the dialysis did for the kidney failure, that is, to become a substitute, a bridge, or a fallback modality. The dream went further. We can make a portable device to remove carbon dioxide, which in turn, enable us to disconnect the respirator (ventilator), eventually close the tracheostomy, and give the patient freedom of speech and ambulation. We will get there.

Respiratory failure is different in many ways than the kidney failure. Patients with emphysema are much older, fragile and are also likely to have associated heart and kidney diseases. With some over simplification it can be said that emphysema, although it is difficult to treat, is eminently a preventable disease, provided we can make the world smoke free.

Emphysema patients are predisposed to having *peptic ulcer disease*. The stomach ulcer can bleed easily on its own or when *anticoagulants or* blood thinning agents are administered to prevent complications of an irregular heart rhythm, or as part of extracorporeal procedure like Hemorespirators.

As it is, there was and still is, substantial doom and gloom attitude about emphysema. That made Hemorespirators not the most ideal technology. It was simple, but not simple enough to be attempted. I should also have put the word "Kissing" in the title of this chapter in the quotes to emphasize the point made by it. *KISS* means *"Keep it simple, stupid!"*

Considering the realities of my life as a research worker, I could not afford to waste my resources of money, equipment, goodwill and a low profile on a half baked technology. I was not interested in just being the first one to try it on a patient to show that it can work. Soon enough it was successfully used in Japan, and I did sincerely congratulate its investigator when I met him many years later.

***

In 1972 I had left the V. A. Hospital after completing my fellowship to join The Coler Memorial Hospital, from where I was permitted to go to the VAH to complete the project Hemorespirators. At Coler I got busy with the BT-PR-EKG studies that ended successfully in the early 1980s. The 1970s also kept me occupied with fighting for the foreign medical graduates (FMG) like myself who were under attacks—unreasonable, according to me—from the organized medicine.

By the late 1970s, my two children were growing up, and I was struggling to impart our language Gujarati, religion Jainism, and our culture to them. I had started to work on several books for that purpose. That venture was quite successful. More information about those publications is in the end pages of this book.

Hemorespirators was not something that I could forget. The question about typhoid fever was a theoretical curiosity, while air in the ABG syringe was incessantly fanning my professional fires.

Every year I did the literature search, that the reader may like to hear about. It is not my purpose here to play the broken record, "Oh, you guys are lucky. You don't know what we had to go through."

What I did go through was not suffering at all, at least it did not feel like it was. The gadgets and facilities that are not discovered or invented yet, cannot make you unhappy by their absence. At best you may dream about them or dream them up and create them. My purpose is to indicate that a research worker has to be prepared to be jack of, or rather almost master of so many things and skills.

The most important skill is to work without proper equipment or facilities, being thankful if one is spared the hostility and violence. Maybe without any rationale, I put my professional fire and the humiliation from the medical profession for being an FMG together, to tell myself, "If you cannot join them, win them." One can try to win them by defeating them or rather win them over, I was willing to take either, preferably the latter.

Coler had not hired me. It was affiliated with New York Medical College which was then at the Flower and Fifth Avenue Hospital in Manhattan, near where Mount Sinai Hospital is today, and was going to move to Westchester. The college had hired me, but it would not let me borrow a book from its library. I mention the college by its name, because if at all, maybe, it was better than most others in that sham and shameful trap called *affiliations*.

Apparently our college did not think I was theirs. Organized medicine including the American Medical Association (AMA), its State branches and the Association of American Medical Colleges (AAMC) were too busy protecting the financial interests of their members to worry about research ideas, or the only available care in the inner city hospitals provided by the FMGs.

ASAIO had more foreigners as members than the American ones, but I could not qualify for their membership. Every year their annual meeting was held during the summer and its transactions were published in a large volume in the fall. I eagerly waited for that to come out, then "buy, borrow or steal" from wherever I could, to stay current and hoping not to see that somebody had published the work that I was hoping and waiting to. That went on for tens of tense years.

In 1975 Dr. Ervido Mejia, a pulmonary specialist like myself joined Coler and began sharing the office with me. That was a two person office, which I had settled in after being moved from offices in one abandoned area to another in various parts of the shrinking hospital.

The office was in a remote wing, euphemistically called just "the South Wing" which housed various labs, X-ray department, an abandoned operating room, and the respiratory therapy services. The chief of the respiratory services, who was an anesthesiologist had her office there, as also did a few pathologists. A room in the abandoned lab was christened "office" before being assigned to me. It had gas lines and burners, full length counter space, with storage cabinets above, and drawers below, as any lab would.

During a subsequent renovation of the area I was asked whether all that should be removed to make more room. I had declined the offer, thinking that it would be impossible to obtain it again, if it would ever be needed. For what, scarcely did I know.

Mejia was from the Dominican Republic and had the temper to go with its stereotype. He was a fine man, good listener and we got to be quite close. I shared my interests and showed him my work. He was fascinated by its potential. He baptized himself, "John the Baptist" in his own words, and I suggested "Sancho Pancha" instead.

In any department conference on dialysis he would invariably ask about using the latter to remove carbon dioxide, the negative answer to which was already known. I had continued to think about simplifying the hemorespirators more. *Only if we could get away* without anticoagulation, or better still without dealing with the blood. But then, that is the only place where carbon dioxide was, or was it?

While I was trying to move that project ahead, I mentioned to Mejia about my work on the books to teach our language, etc., to which he promptly responded, "That's more important than anything else, more needed and more likely to be appreciated in the immediate future." I was already committed to it anyway.

***

Well, the blood carries carbon dioxide and we had to handle the former to extract the latter. Thinking a little more made it obvious that carbon dioxide in its dissolved form, as well as the buffered one, were carried by *plasma*, the liquid, non-cellular part of the blood. Plasma by itself did not clot.

To be correct, plasma devoid of its clotting protein, *fibrinogen,* does not clot. Such plasma is called *serum.*

The only way to get to the serum was to take the blood out, let it clot, then spin it down in a centrifuge to separate its cellular components, leaving behind the serum. So, to escape clotting, you make the blood clot! It made perfect sense. The serum thus obtained would have no carbon dioxide left in solution. Are we going to return it to the patient then? We had to be practical and realistic.

Whenever we talk about "going back to the drawing board," I think of the blackboard in our schools. I prefer to go back to the basics, the basic science that is. The serum must be "True serum" meaning thereby that it is in equilibrium with the blood, that is, the gases are not lost. Accessing it would still be a problem, only a more tangled one.

I kept thinking about the dialysis. We had come that far. The next obvious step was to go for the *peritoneal* dialysis, in which instead of removing the blood (that is, *Hemo dialysis*), purifying and returning it to the body, special water is introduced in the abdomen, around the *viscera* (internal organs), equilibrated its gases and dissolved solutes with the blood in the abdominal wall, then it is drained out and discarded.

Carbon dioxide can easily diffuse out into the fluid and can be removed, but there was a multi-fold problem. One, there is very little carbon dioxide in the dissolved, and therefore, easily removable form. Second, twenty times as much of it is in the buffered form which neither breaks down nor evaporates on being exposed to the room air. Last, unlike other waste products from the dialysis, you cannot just simply discard the buffered gas. This needs to be appreciated clearly.

The massive book from the American Physiological Society, *Handbook of Physiology of Respiration*, taught me the way the existence of the buffered gas was discovered. Investigators collected the dissolved gas which just came out on exposing the *true plasma* to air. Much more carbon dioxide came out when an acid, or the blood was added. Blood was behaving like an acid in this case. This method of adding blood to attack the buffered carbon dioxide appeared to be quite promising.

12. THE RIGHT TO BE WRONG!

When a wrong decision or action suddenly and unexpectedly takes one closer to the goal, it is called serendipity. It plays a major role in research off and on. The erroneous step then becomes a stepping stone.

I was impressed by the idea of liberating carbon dioxide from the bicarb by adding blood. If we take the dialysis fluid from the abdomen, that fluid is expected to be like the *true plasma* without the proteins. It should contain the same amount of carbon dioxide as the patient's blood (Blood-I).

In our schema the fluid coming out of the abdomen goes through a tube to the dialyzer and returns to abdomen, completing the circuit. Another loop from the dialyzer goes into a container of blood (Blood-II) discarded from the blood bank, and returns to the dialyzer. This blood-II can provide the hydrogen ions for removing the bicarbonate.

What a fantastically flawed contraption it was! As described in the physiology book, the blood was behaving like an acid to liberate carbon dioxide from the buffer. The buffer was never a problem, discarding or breaking it down was expected to create one, and I was deliberately embarking upon just that.

It was not difficult to foresee that the method was going to work only temporarily, its performance tapering off as the hydrogen ions in the *Blood-II system* were used up. The blood from blood bank is stored, and it becomes acidic, or loaded with the hydrogen ions, to sustain my delusion.

These hydrogen ions were the ones that I had added, not from the hypothetical patient from whom we wanted remove them. Just about the only thing I was about to prove was that adding an acid to bicarbonate generates carbon dioxide (my stay-at-home wife could have told you that much), destroying the bicarb in the process, and I was the only one in the world to be delighted to rediscover that!

It did get my adrenaline flowing. I designed the apparatus, made a list of materials and equipments that were needed. Fortunately I had no money to buy those things. I did make a few phone calls to get the estimates of the cost. Then on a Friday afternoon, I made the fateful phone call.

That was to a major manufacturer and supplier of renal dialysis equipment. I asked to speak to the manager of their artificial organs division. I wanted to get his opinion about my idea. He was apparently not interested in hearing about the idea, but he went over the laundry list of items that I may need for the experiments and gave me a detailed, more refined and comprehensive version.

Then he suggested that he may be able to send some of the items from his warehouse and indicated that he had a few oxygenators and pumps that were lying around as well and that he was willing to send those also, if I did not mind. They were only for experimental use, not on the patients. No, he did not want me to pay anything and warned me against mentioning his or his company's name anywhere. I had no choice but to agree!

On the following Monday morning, when I reached the hospital and stopped by the department office, I was greeted with unusual warmth and was welcomed by our secretarial staff as if they had been waiting just for me since early morning.

"Thank God, you are finally here!" I heard and looked at my watch. I was not late at all. I did not know what to say.

"What are all these boxes and what to do you want us to with them? They are taking up our entire office!" They were exaggerating only minimally. I carted the 10-15 boxes to my office to my great delight and their relief. I would not try to describe that moment and ruin my memories of it.

I was not unhappy at all that my crazy idea did not quite work, but was rather happy that now at least I could afford to be wrong! That is no small blessing. *If you cannot be wrong, you will have hard time being right.* I informed my benefactor that the Blood-II idea did work, but only minimally. It could not be called a success. However, I had another idea ready and that I had no doubt it would work, because it was simple kindergarten chemistry, so to speak of.

13. THE BLOODLESS REVOLUTION

When our body buffers the acidic carbon dioxide by converting it into the bicarbonate form (see below), a hydrogen ion is set free which is picked up for the time being by hemoglobin. Hydrogen ion is the acid component. In the lungs, the hydrogen ion is picked up, carbon dioxide is unbuffered and is excreted.

Inside the red blood cell

$CO_2 + H_2O = H_2CO_3^-$ (dissolved carbon dioxide)
$H_2CO_3 \longrightarrow H^+ + HCO_3^-$ (buffered carbon dioxide)
H^+ is picked up by Hb   (Hemoglobin)
HCO_3^- moves out of the red blood cell
      as buffered carbon dioxide

The above is reversed in the lungs.

If you simply discard the bicarbonate, the hydrogen ion remains behind and the blood becomes acidic. This is called *metabolic acidosis,* while the retained carbon dioxide that the lungs could not excrete, causes *respiratory acidosis.* Which one is worse is not the question, but both together are the worst. In a patient with respiratory failure and high carbon dioxide level, discarding the bicarbonate is the worst thing one can do.

Not touching it is not an option either. Each 100 ml of the blood contains a mere 2-3 ml of dissolved carbon dioxide and 44 ml of buffered or bicarbonate (-HCO3) carbon dioxide. Note the H in the bicarbonate to understand why it is called *"acid (bi-) carbonate."* Extracting the buffered carbon dioxide would help us lower the flow rate or the amount of blood to be handled to only twentieth that much.

My mission as I could see, was to come up with a way to take out the buffered carbon dioxide and neutralize the hydrogen left behind, at the same time. The former does not give up carbon dioxide when exposed to air. While the dissolved gas would simply escape.

Going back to the early high school days, we can remember that blowing into the lime water makes it turn white. Lime water is $Ca(OH)_2$ and by blowing into it, we add carbon dioxide or CO_2, to produce calcium carbonate or $CaCO_3$.

$$2Ca(OH)_2 + CO_2 = CaCO_3 + H_2O$$

What about the buffered carbon dioxide? It reacts with lime water in the similar way, with a slight difference.

$$2Ca(OH)_2 + (HCO_3{}^-) = CaCO_3 + H_2O + (OH^-)$$
$$2NaOH + (HCO_3{}^-) = Na_2CO_3 + H_2O$$

If we use the sodium hydroxide instead of calcium, no (OH^-) will be released, since sodium (Na^+) is *monovalent*. Both (sodium and calcium) hydroxides are used in the anesthesia machines to absorb the carbon dioxide breathed out by the patient, and to recirculate the very expensive anesthetic gases. They are also used in the spirometers employed to perform the lung function tests.

The hydroxyl ion (OH^-) liberated as above can neutralize the hydrogen to produce water. Mission accomplished! Not so fast. This was tried and had not worked. Dripping a solution of lime water in the dialysis bath worked as it was supposed to. It did combine with both forms of the gas. However, the dialysis membrane got choked up[10] with the impervious calcium carbonate. Adding hydrochloric acid promptly dissolved the precipitate and the dialysis membrane became usable again.

Another one of those "Only if" moments! *Only if we could remove the buffered carbon dioxide and handle the hydrogen ions without clogging up the tubing or the dialyzer!*

I had no trouble procuring the necessary tanks of compressed air and of 10% carbon dioxide (twice the concentration than what we normally breathe out) from the respiratory therapy department next door. I was one of their attending physicians and if needed I could have easily gotten approvals from their Chief and the Chief of Medicine Dr. Wertheimer, who had always supported me. The therapists also gave me a never used carbon dioxide gas analyzer.

One more item still needed was the sodalime granules. I had hoped to get that from the lungs functions lab, but they had run out of them and their next date for ordering the supplies was far in the future. They had enough in their machine. The Chief of the respiratory therapy service, herself an anesthesiologist, Dr. Ana Pla happened to see me and the boxes and came to inquire whether I was moving.

Well, I was on the move, but I needed some help. Coler Hospital had closed for good its surgical suit located two

---

10   Updike SJ, Schults RP, Ghods AJ, Twardowski Z.
        Respiratory gas exchange by hemodialysis.
        Trans Am Soc Artif Int Organs, 1973; 19:529-536.

flights up, many years earlier and Dr. Pla was still coming to supervise the Respiratory Therapy department, to follow the patients on ventilators, and to insert or replace their tracheal tubes. Recalling in time, having seen the granules being used in the anesthesia machines, I asked her whether she could get me some supply of that gas absorber.

She said that was no problem and inquired about the details of my project, which I readily shared with her. I have never been good at keeping secrets unnecessarily. The thought of someone stealing my idea has not been bothersome to me. As it is, the beggars cannot afford to hide their begging bowls, as the Gujarati adage goes.

I had to redefine my mission. Sodalime can substitute for the Blood-II, but what about the clogged tubing? *That was the only problem to be solved to make the system work.* Everything else was in its place. I could use the Blood-II loop to move the reaction away from the "patient."

Dr. Pla returned after 2-3 days according to her part time schedule, looking rather sad. The granules were not expensive at all and if she could not get them, I would have been able to buy them from the market. She did bring the granules, but was afraid that they may not be usable in my circuit.

"Shah, you should read the accompanying pamphlet. I don't know whether they are acceptable. You see, there is lot of water vapor in the expired air returning to our machine, which can dissolve the granules and turn them into a cake. That can block the airflow effectively. To prevent that, this company has come up with water resistant granules that can practically remain soaked in water without disintegrating or caking up. I am afraid...."

"Stop talking, Ana. Can I hug you and give you a kiss?" I grabbed her gently and asked, displaying a behavior absolutely out of my character, professional or personal. She did not mind, but did not understand the reason for my emotional outburst either.

"Yes, they will do. They will do all the work now. There is nothing left for me to do. Ana, don't you see, you just removed my last and the sole remaining hurdle!"

"If you think so." She replied.

Things were moving literally at the speed of light. I spent the following week setting up the circuit a little bit everyday as I got some free time. Thank God, I had kept all those countertops, cabinets, and drawers. Mejia had decided to stay away from there, leaving me alone to concentrate on my work. He always called that room as "Your office" anyway.

The plan was to run the experiment on the following weekend. The circuitry was simple. A bubble oxygenator was to simulate the patient. It was filled with the saline solution through which I ran 10% carbon dioxide gas to simulate retention of carbon dioxide. The gas not absorbed by the saline came out and its concentration was measured by the gas analyzer.

A saline filled tube came out of the bubble oxygenator (the "patient"), went to a dialysis cylinder and returned to the oxygenator. Another loop of tube went from the dialyzer to a container of the Baralyme[11] granules and returned to the dialyzer. This was a "figure of eight, two loops circuit." Only one loop without the dialyzer would have sufficed, but I

---

[11]   Trademark of Chemetron, containing hydroxides of barium, calcium, potassium, and sodium.

wanted to be absolutely certain that no free floating particles clogged up the system. Dialyzer was used only as a filter.

If Baralyme did not remove any carbon dioxide, the "patient" would not pick up any either and the analyzer would display the concentration to be same as at the inlet, that is, 10%. The concentration at the outlet would drop to say 5-6-7% if carbon dioxide was being removed.

What about removing the bicarbonate? I added a measured amount of soda-bicarb ($NaHCO_3$) to the saline. Baralyme also combines with dissolved carbon dioxide to produce bicarbonate.

$$Ca(OH)_2 + HCO_3^- = CaCO_3 + H_2O + (OH^-)$$
$$Ca(OH)_2 + CO_2 = CaCO_3 + H_2O$$
$$(OH^-) + CO2 = HCO_3^-$$
$$(OH^-) + H^+ = H_2O$$

The granules combine with both, the buffered and the dissolved carbon dioxide (top two equations above) to produce calcium carbonate. However, with the buffered carbon dioxide, besides calcium carbonate, it generate a hydroxyle ion.

This system removes both kinds of carbon dioxide, produces a hydroxyle ion to neutralize the hydrogen ions and produce water (equation #4). Hydroxyle ion also reacts with gaseous (dissolved) carbon dioxide to regenerate the bicarbonate (equation #3). This is the beauty of this system. It should be remembered that bicarbonate is not our enemy. It is a friend that brings us lot more carbon dioxide to remove. We do not want to destroy it, just use it to keep carbon dioxide in solution.

Our carrier or transport mechanism is the (OH⁻) ion. It binds to carbon dioxide, forms a bicarbonate, carries it to the Baralyme which precipitates carbon dioxide as calcium carbonate ($CaCO_3$), liberating the (OH⁻) again that can go and bring more carbon dioxide.

This (OH⁻) comes from the bicarb that we had added to neutralize the acidic saline solution, and some more. In real life, it can come from the patient, although I would prefer to provide it myself, so that the patient does not lose any of his or her own essential bicarbonate.

I ran the experiment for maybe 3 hours. It showed that the system could function without deterioration for at least two or more hours. It was easy to run. There were no leakage or pressure problem. Wet Baralyme does have a chalk like odor, and it does get warm, as an added advantage.

The rate of removal of carbon dioxide by this system is dependent upon the fluid flow rate of both pumps, one in each loop, gas flow rate at the inlet and the concentration of the bicarbonate in the system. All these variables are controllable by the investigator and hence, the system does not appear to be limited in any way.

The detailed results became available over the next couple of days, but on that weekend day I of course called Usha to give her the good news. Then called the head nurse of the respiratory care unit Ms. Terry Mosler, R.N. who was a wonderful team member to work with and with whom I had gone over the intricacies of the acid-base physiology. She was working that day and she came over right away.

I showed her the experimental setup and explained what she was looking at. She calmly said that she believed me, that she could see my uncharacteristic excitement and was quite happy to be invited to share it. Oh! Only if it was easier to live with such *Eureka* moments!

On Monday, I practically ran the experiment again from scratch for Mejia to see it first hand. He was highly excited and he congratulated me on that much awaited moment. Over the following week I ran the experiment several times to obtain more data and to reproduce the data that I already had.

During that week I called my benefactor who had made the experiments possible, to report my success with the new method. He said that he had never doubted that it could be done. When he had offered the equipment, etc., I had had the feeling that he had not heard anything I had tried to tell him about the idea or my plans to bring it to fruition. So, what was behind his generosity?

He confided in me that many years earlier, when he had joined the company as the chief of its artificial organs division, his mission was to make the peritoneal dialysis usable for removing carbon dioxide. He knew that it should be and would be possible to do so, but he could not achieve it. When he heard the purpose of what I was trying to do, that was enough for him. He was sure, I would vindicate him.

He did not share with me the details of various methods that he had tried. Peritoneal dialysis thus modified looks simple enough to carry out, and it really is so, but there was an enormous theoretical background to support it. There were several serious issues that had to be resolved to make the process practical. The biggest one was to extract continuously the buffered carbon dioxide without causing acidosis. That was finally done.

The dialysis project had a code name in my files, *PR,* for *peritoneal respirizer.* Let me summarize what was done and what was achieved:

1. A *modified* circuit of peritoneal dialysis was used.
2. *Recirculation* of peritoneal fluid was the major modification. This was done to avoid affecting any small or large molecules from being exchanged, except for carbon dioxide.
3. No dialysis as we know occurs at the low flow rates employed, and the recirculation does not favor any exchange across the membrane.
4. This model resembles "tidal volume" dialysis, in which only a fraction of the fluid volume is treated in the circuit, while most of it remains in the abdominal cavity, getting equilibrated with the body. The term *tidal dialysis* was not known at the time of the experiments and was going to be coined a decade hence.
5. No tubing got clogged up.
6. No acid administration was required to unclog the tubing.
7. Both, dissolved and buffered carbon dioxide were removed.
8. Bicarbonate carbon dioxide was removed, hydroxyl ion was produced. Hydroxyl ion reacted with carbon dioxide to regenerate the bicarb.
9. No bicarb was discarded, destroyed, or removed.
10. Hydroxyl ion acted as a carrier to transport carbon dioxide as bicarbonate.
11. Initially bicarbonate was added to prevent the destruction of that of the "patient."

12. All variables affecting the removal of carbon dioxide were controllable by the investigator.
13. No blood was used, hence no anticoagulation was needed.
14. It seems feasible to prepare a *portable* peritoneal dialysis model to wean the emphysema patients off respirators and to restore their freedom of speech and mobility.
15. Working on the above is recommended for the future.
16. Baralyme has a chalky odor, which is easily tolerable in a well ventilated room.
17. Baralyme does get warm to touch, and that may be able to counter the feared heat loss caused by exposing the fluids to room temperature.

14. "MY DAD LIVES ON CARBON DIOXIDE!"

My daughter Manisha was a teenager when she made the above observation. From 1971 through 1987 I was breathing only carbon dioxide. After the success of the dialysis experiment, I had started to breathe oxygen again, except when my breath was taken away by the events that followed.

A few days before the experiment, I had sent some material about the Hemorespirator project to Dr. Landé, the inventor of the membrane lung that I had used, to request him to sponsor my abstract to the ASAIO. He had shown willingness to do so. I called him again to inform him of the new development, which he received with interest, and added that he was not much into the dialysis area of the field.

With an unusual daring on my part, I asked him whether he would be kind enough to extend the same favor to another abstract, that describing the modified peritoneal dialysis. He agreed to look at it, and I sent him both abstracts by regular mail. He sponsored both and forwarded them to the ASAIO before the rapidly approaching deadline for submission. Both were published in the ASAIO Abstracts[12], the Hemorespirators one after 15 years, and the dialysis one only within three or four months after the experiments. Talk about rapid publication!

Hemorespirator paper was published at the end of 1985. Then I was allowed to become a member of the ASAIO,

---

[12] Correction of experimental hypercapnia and hypoxemia with membrane lungs.
ASAIO Abstracts. 1985. 14; p. 67.

Chemical extraction of carbon dioxide via modified peritoneal dialysis. A model simulation.
ASAIO Abstracts. 1985. 14; p. 67.

even though I had only one such paper on my name. I guess they must have counted two abstracts also to qualify me. I had had attended the annual ASAIO meetings several times between 1971 and 1986. As I was not a member, I had to pay a higher registration fee, but that was paid for by the college, as mandatory continuing medical education (CME).

It was always a pleasure to attend the ASAIO meetings. Their atmosphere was professional, awe inspiring and yet collegial. Great inventors and investigators from all over the world came there and joined everybody else at the breakfast, lunch, and dinner tables. People were friendly, helpful and down to earth. Many if not most were foreigners and a good many of them had only a minimal acquaintance with the English language.

Somehow, even after I became a member, my name always seemed to disappear from their members' list. I always ended up paying the nonmembers' rates for the registration. Twice I wrote to the presidents of the ASAIO, to no avail. This apparently did not succeed in taking away my excitement and delight at being able to be there. *That was the only time and place when I felt that I was part of an international professional academic brotherhood.*

***

One Italian group lead by Gattinoni had started publishing articles on low blood flow removal of carbon dioxide, but their blood flow rates were hardly low in comparison with what we had used in Hemorespirators. They were using oxygen also. During the discussion of one of their papers, Dr. Kolobov from the NIH, who was collaborating with them mentioned that they were surprised to see the oxygen level improve. I patted myself on the back for predicting that in my protocol, when I was a second year fellow, maybe 15 years earlier.

It seemed that we were quite close to one another in our goal, but were approaching it from opposite sides. I could not think of any reason why they would use such high blood flow rates and a high oxygen concentration for removing carbon dioxide. I wrote a letter to Dr. Gattinoni.

In the subsequent meeting of the ASAIO in New York, I heard a member of the Gattinoni group present their findings. I met him and he informed me that he had seen the letter and that it was discussed by them. Another investigator presented findings of a controlled experiment to show that there was no survival benefit with the Italian group's method of removing carbon dioxide. I joined the discussion and reported on the results of the dialysis experiments.

A few months later I got an invitation to go to Marburg in Germany (West Germany, then) to present the results of my experiments. The Powerpoint was not there yet. As usual, I prepared the illustrations manually, photographed them and printed them for possible publication. For the presentation at the conference, I prepared two sets of Polaroid slides with blue background setting off white letters, quite familiar to the old timers.

My wife Usha and I were the guests of the Marburg University for three days. Their hospitality of all the attendees was lavish. My presentation was for half an hour followed by a question-answer period, quite long for an international meeting. I met the Gattinoni group, the Japanese investigator who had had used the ECMO for respiratory failure and Dr. Kolobov from the NIH, the leading pediatric ECMO giant Dr. Bartlett, and a few others.

Results of the modified dialysis experiments were published[13] as a paper in the ASAIO Journal. My presentation in Marburg was published as a book chapter[14] in their transactions.

***

On the job front back home in New York, even the sham affiliation with the college was going to end, with the City moving towards disaffiliations. The college hired back only one physician that it had dumped on us years earlier, but none of us. The Dean to be, from another affiliated hospital expressed his inability to hire us for want of vacancy, when his own hospital had run an ad to recruit the faculty in that very day's New York Times.

Disgusting as all this was, my dealing with the Office of the Research Administration in Westchester, NY and with their animal lab in the city were productive. The new Chairman of the Pulmonary Service, whom I met to discuss the possibility of furthering my work, frankly told me that he was under strict orders not to deal with anybody from Coler.

I was in number two position in my department, but was worried that any cost cutting measures would find it attractive to eliminate my position. Research wise, there was

---

[13]   An in vitro model for chemical extraction of carbon dioxide via modified peritoneal dialysis.
ASAIO Transactions. 1988; 34: 112-115.

[14]   Extraction of carbon dioxide via modified peritoneal dialysis.
P. 221-27, in
Neonatal and adult respiratory failure:
Mechanisms and treatments. In
Gille JP, editor,
Editions Scientifiques Elsevier (Paris), for the
Commission of the European Communities, 1989.

no hope of getting anything substantial done in that environment. I decided to go to the ASAIO meeting scheduled to be held in Reno, Nevada. I knew that would be the last conference to be paid for by the college.

The flight to Reno left New York very early in the morning and I had to get up a few hours still earlier. I took some coffee at home, then in the plane a couple of times. In Reno it was still afternoon and the meeting was in progress. I took some more coffee and sat through it.

My interest was in the next day's program. On my way to my hotel room I found out about the ASAIO president's welcome party for the new members, slated for that evening at 9 p.m. I took still some more coffee and finally *went* to sleep, but I could not. Every little noise startled me, soon I was afraid of a break-in and found myself sitting on the edge of the bed guarding my room with nothing of any value to anybody else in it. I diagnosed my hyper-vigilant state as *caffeine intoxication.* Finally I fell asleep to wake up after the morning session, which I wanted to attend, was over.

I dragged myself to the elevator bank on the 27th floor to go to the conference. The elevator came down to my floor bringing 3-4 doctors with the ASAIO badge affixed to their lapel. I entered the elevator and greeted them, introducing myself. The leader of the group responded,

"Oh, yes. Dr. Shah! We know you very well. We are the members of your fan club!" I wondered whether that was a joke.

"I am indeed honored, but can you please enlighten me?"

"Well, I am Dr. Michael Klein. We heard you in Marburg and loved your presentation."

"Yours was the bloody only one that made some sense," someone added. I soaked it in. Dr. Klein's name did not ring any bells. I apologized. He asked me whether I was planning to attend a certain afternoon session that he was going to chair. I had, indeed, planned to attend that. He asked me not to change my plans, then added that he "needed" me there.

That session was on artificial lungs, mostly for the open heart surgery. Hardly any group was working on perfecting the former for treating respiratory failure, at least, not in the U.S.A. I commented on one of the papers presented there and was going to go back to my seat, when Dr. Klein asked me to stay at the microphone to answer a couple of other questions he was going to raise.

Another paper was by a Dr. Steven Nolte from Germany, on the *feasibility of using* a low blood flow ECMO for removing carbon dioxide—something that I had been working on for the past 15 years and had already achieved that experimentally three four years earlier. I was not apprehensive at all, because I was way ahead.

When Dr. Klein invited comments and looked at me, I avoided his gaze, finding it too embarrassing and impolite to our overseas guest to pour cold water on his work. Then Dr. Klein requested the pioneer and the leading authority on the pediatric ECMO, Dr. Bartlett, for his comments. He was the most appropriate and knowledgeable person familiar with my work to remark on that paper.

"We, here in the United States have lately been exploring a new modality, that of modified peritoneal dialysis for removing carbon dioxide." Dr. Bartlett began.

Such moments come only rarely in one's life. It was a trivial event of no larger significance. However, for me it was something that I had waited for, all my life. I knew what Dr.

Bartlett meant when he said, "We." He was referring to me, a poor little FMG, with supposedly poor medical and English language skills, invading the US to snatch away jobs and patients from the battle worn American doctors!

I was as if, carrying the American flag in that international prestigious body, when almost everybody else had abandoned working on artificial lungs for an irreversible disease like emphysema, as a lost cause. Like that Japanese soldier, I had kept on fighting his Emperor's war (WW-II), unaware that the latter was over long ago.

Eventually I did add my comments gently and carefully. Dr. Nolte did not look disturbed at all. He appeared to have been expecting that all along. After the meeting we lingered to meet one another. He introduced me to his wife, who told me, with her husband translating, that ever since the Marburg meeting he had been talking to her about a Dr. Shah from the US, who had already done the work.

Then he went on to offer an apology for his inability to do anything about the acceptance of his paper by the ASAIO. The irony was, my paper had seen the daylight in his native place. Apparently, there was enough carbon dioxide around for both of us to breathe comfortably.

I was at the top of my world, and that world was being turned upside down! All those delightful cordial and collegial moments were not going to survive once they reached New York. The affiliation was dissolved. My job was likely to be phased out. I could not afford to take any chances. I resigned and moved to a State mental health hospital on an adjacent island, where my boss had moved three years earlier. When the world around us is going mad, what could be saner than moving into a mental hospital?

15. "YEARNING TO BREATHE FREE"

The Hemorespirators and the modified peritoneal Dialysis, both projects were conceived with the intent to help patients with emphysema and respiratory failure associated with retention of carbon dioxide. Both sets of experiments consisted of raising the blood level of carbon dioxide, to be then corrected by experimental means. Such rapid elevation of carbon dioxide is called an *acute* rise.

Both our approaches worked well with the acute rise, which is quite drastic. ECMO was successfully tried in one such patient in Japan, it has been tried for respiratory resuscitation (like CPR, in the U.S.A.). However, it remains too complex to be put in common use. Long standing elevation of carbon dioxide is called the *chronic* rise, and such patients are generally on the long term respiratory support being provided through ventilators.

The chronic rise is found in relatively stable patients, not in immediate danger of dying. They usually have a *tracheostomy*—a hole in the wind pipe, below the voice box—through which passes a four inch long plastic tube into the upper airways. Its outer end is connected to a ventilator, and an airtight circuit is ensured.

No air is permitted to go through the voice box and the vocal cords situated above it, by using an inflated balloon, thereby making it impossible for the patient to talk. This is very frustrating for the patient. Being unable to verbalize, being afraid of the machine's stopping at any time, being literally tied down to the latter around the clock, with no hope of ever getting away from it, makes the patient miserable.

These patients were the targeted recipients of the modified dialysis system. The peritoneal approach leaves the patient's neck untouched, and his or her speech is not impaired—a major and worthwhile gain in itself. Changing the peritoneal tubes is not likely to generate as much apprehension as changing a tracheostomy tube.

Moreover, the dialysis system can operate on battery powered pumps, and it may allow the patient to ambulate to the bathroom, then the day room, and then maybe, to the board room of the corporate office where (s)he worked! Let us review the factors that make this possible.

Hypothesis:
1. We have demonstrated the feasibility of very low blood flow Hemorespirators, using compressed air to remove carbon dioxide, correcting the Ventilatory Deficit to provide *para-corporeal* ECMO support
2. Peritoneal fluid is similar to plasma, it is "true plasma," in its *dissolved* and *buffered* carbon dioxide content that is identical to that of the blood, making both of them accessible for extraction by chemical means employing calcium hydroxide.
3. Carbon dioxide is precipitated as carbonate with calcium hydroxide reacting with either dissolved or buffered carbon dioxide.
4. Buffered carbon dioxide, when thus precipitated, liberates a hydroxyl ion, which can
    I.   Neutralize hydrogen ion held by the hemoglobin to form water, or
    II. Can combine with carbon dioxide to regenerate the bicarbonate.

5. Thus, no bicarbonate is lost but it is regenerated, with the hydroxyl ion acting as a carrier of bicarbonate carbon dioxide.

6. No blood, acid, or anticoagulant drug is used in the system

7. Recirculation dialysis is employed. No conventional dialysis of solutes takes place. No water gain or loss is generated. Only carbon dioxide is extracted.

8. Emphysema patients can accommodate a liter or more of extra water in their peritoneal cavity. We add bicarbonate to prime the system, rather than risk losing the patient's bicarbonate.

9. We may need to *clear* only two glassfuls of peritoneal fluid of carbon dioxide every minute, containing about 200 ml, which is the resting total production of carbon dioxide. Far less than that may be needed to be extracted.

10. *Barium Hydroxide has been used as a rodent poison,* and we may have to use the calcium salt or to check with the manufacturer about the toxicity. Baralyme is being safely used in rebreathing circuits of anesthesia machines, though.

11. With retention of carbon dioxide, as it occurs in patients with one kind of emphysema, CO_2 *content* in the peritoneal fluid increases, making the system self controlling to some extent.

12. This system of respiratory support allows respiratory rehab to strengthen the respiratory muscles simultaneously.

13. Tracheostomy may soon be removed or kept only for the *bronchial toilet.* In either case, patient's speech can be restored to improve the quality of life.

14. Ambulation can be attempted gradually and progressively to facilitate vocational training and employment.
15. This radically different method only superficially resembles conventional renal peritoneal dialysis, since most of the principles and actions used go against the fundamentals of peritoneal dialysis, e.g., recirculation, absence of transfer of solutes and water, and extraction of carbon dioxide with a chemical.
16. There are ways to play with the settings of the volume respirators to create leaks intentionally to permit the patient to talk. I have used this without any problem except objections from a new therapist.
17. Other methods like the tracheal suctioning (to be presented later under "Why do patients with tracheostomy like to have it suctioned?") that the patients with tracheostomies seem to like, need to be explored to see whether a new modality can be developed from that.
18. Despite the doom and gloom attitude prevalent regarding emphysema, a lot can still be achieved.

Since I left Coler Hospital in 1988, I have been trying hard to further this method of recirculation, tidal volume dialysis system with no success. The system is like a ripe fruit, ready to be plucked and enjoyed to a great delight of many.

OVERLOOKED MIRACLE CURES?

16. PHENYTOIN FOR SMOKING CESSATION

My battle was against the aftermaths of emphysema and despite the success of the Hemorespirator and the peritoneal dialysis, I could see that it was far more effective to prevent it. I was wondering why people would smoke, albeit in a relatively smaller proportion than before, even when they were knowledgeable about its dangers.

Survival of emphysema patients was at my heart, but my own survival was taking up my mind. Manhattan Psychiatric Center (MPC) in 1988 was not what it is in 2011. When I joined it I could not believe or even imagine that even in America, a hospital—albeit mental—can be as pathetic as that.

Old wards with dark long hallways, peeling paint applied repeatedly over ancient wooden and metal doors fitting poorly, rattling and permitting the gusty wind to produce an eerie sound, all created a depressing atmosphere. The ventilation was poor and large but dirty glass windows divided into several horizontal panels with five smaller windows each felt confining and suffocating.

As if that was not enough, cigarette smoking among its inhabitants and staff members was rampant. Smoking was almost a necessity to help both of them keep their cool, at least for a while. To be a nonsmoker there was as easy as remaining a virgin in a brothel. It was not an inviting place for a nonsmoker specialist in diseases of the chest.

I was part of the Medical Services of MPC, to take care of medical complications and consequences of mental disease, epilepsy, drug addiction, uncontrolled sexual activity—consensual and otherwise, violence amongst patients or directed towards the staff, severe side effects of essential drug therapy and obesity. The AIDS was more common in such hospitals and correctional facilities, or prisons. There was a very thin line between those two.

Most patients then were generally healthy, medically speaking, making it possible for one medical doctor to cover two psychiatric wards, each of which had at least two psychiatrists. On my very first day there, I went back to my chief to tell him that there was no way I could *see* patients or anything else. The wards were so full of thick smoke that I doubt whether one could cut it even with a knife.

Cutting the red tape and age old traditions was difficult still. Smoking was supposed to be the patients' inalienable right, never mind that it was not right for them to smoke. It was a lollipop to keep them quiet. I had to voluntarily keep myself imprisoned in my office, going to the treatment room to see patients only when needed, or to go to the common hall—called a *dayroom*, where patients spent their free time, which encompassed all their waking hours.

The smoke did not clear, nor did I get used to it. It was too obvious not to see. What struck me was that there was no clear explanation why they smoked and why so much. There were anecdotal comments blaming the heavy smoking on poor upbringing, lawless mentality, criminal tendency, boredom, laziness, addiction, oral stage of sexuality and so on. The staff smoked because a few of them were ex mental patients themselves and because the rest of the country smoked.

One did not have to study pulmonary medicine to know that in the general population, the prevalence of smoking was 30% and that had come down to 25% by the late 1980s. Compared to that national average, 75% of the patients in MPC were smokers. Being a research worker all my life and being just curious, I thought of studying the smoking behavior of the psychiatric patients.

Where should I begin? It was not possible to study all smokers. They could be subdivided but, along which lines? Women were also smoking and their proportion of smokers was apparently the same as that of men. Selecting a particular diagnostic group was not practical because *schizophrenia* and *bipolar disorder* were the major groups. It was frustrating and I was not able to see my mission clearly, literally and figuratively.

During my residency training in the late 1960s, I had received free copies of two hard cover books from a Jack Dryfus, drawing attention to the anti-seizures or anti-epilepsy drug phenytoin sodium (Dilantin, Parke-Davis & Company). The smaller book was entitled, "A Remarkable Medicine Has Been Overlooked!" It was not, I thought. That was the best selling drug for epilepsy and a few other conditions.

The other was a three or four times bigger companion volume listing 3500 or so references culled from the medical literature, according to its compiler. I had no reason to look at the references and I had not.

The book on phenytoin was small, easy to read and was about the drug that I was quite familiar with. It seemed to me that the author, whom I knew nothing about in my those early days in the US, was advocating some new uses for the drug. I was too busy getting my medical license, and clearing the board exam, to read it.

A few days later I thought of getting rid of it, but I had not yet acquired the wasteful habit of throwing away brand new books or newspapers without even looking at them cursorily. Even today, I cannot do that. My last subscription to the home delivery of New York Times was more than 15 years ago. I now subscribe to their on-line edition.

The books stayed with me for years and years, moving with me from hospital to hospital as I moved. A couple of times I did put them in the garbage, heeding the advice, "If you did not use it in ten years, you don't need it!" However, before the trash was picked up, I retrieved them.

If I recall correctly, I had planned to work on one of my research manuscripts, but at home we had received some unexpected and long term guests. Therefore, I decided to read it whenever I could, when the guests were busy doing their things. If I was going to read it at all, then that was the time.

Dryfus did not appear to be a physician. He was in the stock market. He had been diagnosed to have been depressed. He felt that all cells of his brain were firing simultaneously, making it impossible for him to concentrate. He recalled one of his cousins with epilepsy which was treated with phenytoin to "calm down her nerves."

He had persuaded his psychiatrist friend to prescribe phenytoin for him to make his nerves behave in an orderly manner. Medically speaking, the logic was poor. However, the psychiatrist had obliged. Dryfus felt miraculously better, against all expectations. He tried to convince the medical and the government hierarchy including a couple of Presidents, to no avail.

Lot of water had gone under the bridge since I had received the books and read them 20 years later. I did know by then that Mr. Dryfus was the successful founder of the major financial house of Dryfus. Being a man of strong determination and means to match it, he had self published the books and sent them free of charge to all doctors, just when I had joined their ranks as a neophyte intern.

Phenytoin was also used to treat irregular heart rhythm, I knew and had used it for that purpose. Phenytoin acts like the president of a meeting where everybody is trying to talk simultaneously. (S)he uses the gavel to stop everyone from talking, she waits for complete silence and then permits one of them to speak.

The same is done by phenytoin to all cells of heart or brain firing at the same time. They are all quietened down, thereby wiping the slate clean. Then an orderly firing of electrical discharges resumes, allowing the heart or the brain to function efficiently. A feeling of calm is thus generated.

Reading that was the *Gotcha!* moment. If phenytoin induces the calm, that may be a good substitute for smoking by the patients in MPC. There are many real and presumed factors that can induce smoking behavior. Searching for the calm is one of them. A hypothesis began to take shape.

Hypothesis:
1. Those patients who were receiving phenytoin for any reason at all, would be less likely to be smokers,
2. If they did smoke, they were likely to smoke less,

3. The calming effect of phenytoin is most likely to be centrally mediated, that is, a direct action on the brain, and if that is so,

4. Phenytoin would be expected to remove the craving for smoking cigarettes. Many smokers, especially women, are afraid to quit for the fear of subsequent weight gain. The weight gain occurs thanks to the craving for cigarettes, which if left unappeased leads to overeating as a substitute. If there is no craving left, then there would not be any reason to overeat and,

5. Patients who are receiving phenytoin would be expected to weigh less than the smokers and the non-smoker control group of patients.

If the hypothesis turns out to be valid, the reader can easily see why phenytoin would make an ideal smoking cessation therapy. Smoking is an addiction. Any attempt to quit cold turkey is met with severe craving. Many have successfully quit in this fashion. Like smoking, eating and sex are also addictive. Dryfus' book mentioned using phenytoin successfully to treat unstable diabetes, and violence and other behavior problems in prison inmates and in the general population.

My assignment also included going to the special ward for the extremely violent patients. I was getting progressively more interested in that aspect of psychiatric problems. However, one needs to have more intimate knowledge of the problem to work on it. Therefore, that aspect of the possible phenytoin treatment had to wait.

Although MPC then outwardly looked like an ancient and down right primitive institution straight from the dark ages, but it was the most highly computerized facility I had come across. Computers were in common use in all departments. They were not yet to be found in all medical physicians' offices, but senior psychiatrists, department heads and various administrative offices were equipped with them. When I left it after 15 years of service, all doctors, and nurses' stations had a desk top computer work station.

The new Chief of the Medical Services, Dr. Harold Ratner, was a computer genius. With his help I was able to get a printout from the pharmacy, of all patients who were receiving phenytoin. A list of patients residing in MPC used to come out every week. Using the relational databases with Dr. Ratner's help, in a matter of a few hours, I was able to get all the desired information on those patients.

The list of patients made it easy to select age and sex matched *control* patients who were not receiving phenytoin, from the same wards. Then I went to those wards to get the information on body weights and smoking habits of patients. In mental hospitals, the inpatients are not permitted to carry a matchbox with them but had to ask a staff member to help them light up a cigarette. Therefore, the staff knew every patient's smoking habit in great detail, including his or her getting violent on not getting a cigarette.

The findings validated the hypothesis. The 25 patients receiving phenytoin for various diseases, were less likely to be smokers, if they did smoke, they were likely to smoke less and as a group, and they weighed less. All results were statistically significant at 5% level.

The findings were published[15] as a letter to the editor and then as a full paper[16] in the New York State Journal of Medicine. That is the reason, I am not reporting here the findings in detail.

***

Among the 3500 or so citations in Dryfus' companion volume, there was not a single reference to the effect of phenytoin on the smoking behavior. That was surprising. However, a research worker learns early enough not to be surprised with anything. As a corollary to that, (S)he also learns not to assume anything.

I casually dialed Mr. Dryfus' office after looking up the phone number for the Dryfus Medical Foundation and asked to speak to Mr. Dryfus. I do not know how many such crazy calls his secretary gets every year, but she politely conveyed that she was not going to put me through.

She wanted to know the nature of my business. I told her that I wanted to discuss a medical matter with him, but that did not cut any ice either. Finally, I started to tell her that I had done some work on Dilantin, the name he had used in his book, when suddenly a male voice cut in, "Jack Dryfus here!"

I quickly told him why I was calling. He listened with great interest. After giving him the results of my study, I

---

15   Shah BS, Harold Ratner, M.D.
      Phenytoin and smoking.
      New York State J Med. 1992; 71-72.

16   Shah BS, Harold Ratner, M.D.
      Anti-convulsant drugs, smoking, and body weights in psychiatric
      inpatients.
      New York State J Med. 1993; 16-17.

asked him whether he had come across any such thing after he had published the book. He had not.

He asked me to continue the conversation, but mentioned that he would love to have the Medical Director of his private medical foundation to hear what I was telling him. He added that he was not trying to cut me short, then continued to talk on the phone for about three-fourth of an hour. Finally, he asked the secretary to make an appointment for my wife Usha and myself to meet him and Dr. Smith in his office.

A few days later we went to meet Mr. Dryfus in his eleventh floor penthouse office next to the Plaza hotel, facing the Central Park to the North. He himself offered us the coffee on an ornate silver service. Then he asked me to tell Dr. Smith about my work. Mr. Dryfus listened intently, as if he had never heard that before, emphasizing a few points that I did not.

They offered us a set of their books. Although I had the books I took them and asked Dr. Smith and Mr. Dryfus to autograph them. Mr. Dryfus thanked us for coming over and I thanked him for having us there.

"Call me *Jack.*" He said, after hearing me say *Mr. Dryfus* several times.

"No way! You will have to forgive me for that." I politely declined.

"Why not, may I ask?" He persevered by asking a rhetorical question. He had been to India and he probably knew very well that it would be the height of disrespect for me to do so. Then I took the middle path, addressing him as Mr. Dryfus and referring to him in the third person as Jack.

Then I apologized for carrying *the coal to Newcastle* by talking to him about Dilatin. He matched that with his wisdom, saying, "You can never light fire under a turtle. A fire is lit under you and you are running as fast as you can. I wish you all the best." He started after Dr. Smith had left.

I asked him about how his campaign to popularize Dilantin was going over all these years. He was not happy with the way it was. He informed me that he had more favorable reception in Russia, China and India, as opposed to right here at home in the U.S. He wondered, why.

"Mr. Dryfus (He did not correct me), you are the head of a major capitalist corporation, so I am a bit uncomfortable telling this. Those countries are not capitalist. They don't have much money, but they do generally hold education to be almost holy, not to be tainted with money. Pursuit of truth and knowledge there does not always depend on money alone."

He told me about his trying to draw attention to Dilantin which was pigeonholed in treatment of epilepsy and practically nothing else. Its manufacturer, Parke-Davis had not spent a penny on Dilantin in recent years, he had mentioned in his book. The Food and Drugs Administration (FDA), medical journals and the Presidents—He had met three of them, Nixon, Carter and Reagan—to no avail.

Pulling out a photograph of himself and Mr. Reagan, he said, "This is about the all that came out of the meeting." Then he added, "Do you know, the business of medicine does not even have a receptionist? If you want to tell them something, you won't know where to go."

"You are speaking from experience, Mr. Dryfus. Well, for my part, I *have* listened to you and have benefitted from it. Let me ask you, looking back, do you recall anytime when you might have witnessed the antismoking effect of Dilantin?" I continued to refer to phenytoin by its trade name, as he had done in his book and during our meeting. There was no reference to that in his book.

"There was, come to think of it. Once when I was playing bridge at the Cavendish Club, a friend dropped by at our table. He was a chain smoker and probably had emphysema, too. He was out of breath, which he used to do often. I was always carrying Dilantin in my pocket and offered it freely to anybody who would need it and take it."

"I gave him maybe 50 mg of Dilantin (the anti-epilepsy dose is 300 mg per day, and it takes several hours to days to work). He returned after a couple of hours, feeling much better, which was not surprising. That he had not smoked a cigarette during *that long time*, was surprising. Maybe I should have paid more attention to that." He concluded.

After a couple of weeks I read in the New York Times that the financial house of Dryfus was sold for 386 million dollars.

17. PHENYTOIN FOR VIOLENT BEHAVIOR

Using phenytoin therapy to control violent behavior in prisons, and in mental health facilities is an interesting possibility to explore. There were many references in Dryfus' book on this topic. However, I had not yet picked up that aspect of phenytoin to do any serious thinking through, and I will leave it at that.

18. PHENYTOIN AS AN IDEAL WEIGHT-LOSS DRUG

In the preceding chapters we glossed over the possible role of phenytoin in management of violence and we briefly went over the lower body weight of the patients who were receiving phenytoin. The latter is an anti-epileptic drug working directly on the brain (that is, *centrally*) and would be expected to remove the craving for smoking cigarettes.

Many smokers, especially women are afraid to quit for the fear of subsequent weight gain which occurs thanks to the craving for cigarettes. When left unappeased, the latter leads to overeating as a substitute. Any attempt to quit smoking cold turkey is met with severe craving. Many have tolerated the craving and quit successfully in this fashion.

Like smoking, eating and sex are addictive, too. If there is no craving left, then there would not be any need to overeat and therefore, patients who are receiving phenytoin would be expected to weigh less than the smokers, those ex-smokers who had quit smoking in another way, and non-smokers.

As expected according to the hypothesis, patients receiving phenytoin did weigh less. The weight gain associated with quitting smoking was apparently being curtailed or neutralized by phenytoin. This is important especially for women smokers, who would rather prefer to lose the battle against smoking than the "battle of the bulge," by choosing to continue smoking over gaining weight.

This finding can be extended to lead us into a fertile field of study. Can phenytoin be used as a weight loss drug? The answer appears to be affirmative. Why belabor this point which is so obvious by now? Because it is obviously not clearly appreciated. Its implications are far more diverse and significant.

Obesity is literally a *growing* problem in America. We do not need statistics to make that point. Diet, exercise, drugs, everything have been around for a long time, together with controversies surrounding them. Even if one can lose only a few pounds, keeping them off for long is not easy. "Yo-yo" dieting is not helpful, and it may be quite harmful.

I know a couple of people whose weigh seems to change over the course of the year from being sickly thin to looking like a balloon, like phases of the moon. In extreme cases, and in not so extreme cases also, reducing the size of the stomach, or bypassing a major part of it surgically have been done. These procedures have a high incidence of complications, including death.

The so called diet drugs themselves are not palatable or easy to take. They cause dryness of mouth, eye problems, prostate problems, severe and fatal heart complications, and what not. Some are fraught with seizures. There is an obvious need for a good diet drug.

A good or ideal diet drug should be effective, safe, easy to take, and must address the root cause of becoming overweight. Phenytoin has been around for 75 years, and doctors know how to handle it. In the dosage used to treat seizures, say 300 mg per day, it is not free from side effects, mainly anemia and gum disease.

Recently, occurrence of suicidal ideations and attempts have been reported in patients taking conventional doses of some weight loss drugs, as well as in patients taking phenytoin.

That was the dose MPC patients were appropriately getting. However, based on Dryfus' observations, for treating conditions other than seizures the necessary dose of phenytoin may be as low as 100 mg daily or maybe, still less. That can avoid many side effects.

Most other diet drugs attempt to curb the appetite or make the food unpalatable by causing a dry mouth. Phenytoin works centrally removing the craving and inducing a calm, without leaving any feeling of deprivation. Our study patients had not been trying to lose weight, based on what we do know about them. If someone *is* motivated to lose weight, the results might be even better.

For the same reason, keeping the pounds off should be easier with phenytoin treatment. A *maintenance therapy*, probably in smaller or less frequent dosage may suffice for that. Phenytoin appears to be a promising diet drug by way of its safety profile, effectiveness in inducing weight loss and helping to keep the pounds off without making the individual miserable, and hence, it is worth a trial.

I had inquired and collected information about doing a clinical drug trial. The FDA has an imposing, intimidating, and dense application form for granting a waiver for an experimental drug. I suppose, since phenytoin is not exactly a new or experimental drug anyway, a simpler application may suffice. Let us formally state the hypothesis.

Hypothesis:
1. Phenytoin treatment was observed to have been associated with a relatively lower body weight.
2. Its action is assumed to be central, based on what is known about it.

3. It is known to curtail craving and induce a calm. This may have replaced the potential weight gain in non-smokers and those who smoked less, with a lower weight.

4. These findings can possibly be extended to general population, including smoker and nonsmoker obese people.

5. A lower dose than that required to control seizures, in the range of 50-250 mg daily may be adequate.

6. Side effects from phenytoin in that dose may be less likely and less severe.

7. Phenytoin may be a motivational drug, too. Patients in my study[17] were not getting it explicitly for smoking cessation or weight reduction, and yet they had achieved both.

8. Phenytoin may be good for crisis intervention, to curb appetite while one is attending a party, etc., since it is known to work quite rapidly to *induce calm*.

9. Phenytoin is expected to be a good maintenance therapy as well to keep the weight low.

10. Phenytoin seems to be the ideal drug for fighting our national epidemic of obesity and diabetes, with their consequences.

---

17   Shah BS, Harold Ratner, M.D.
Phenytoin and smoking.
New York State J Med. 1992; 71-72.

Shah BS, Harold Ratner, M.D.
Anti-convulsant drugs, smoking, and body weights in
Psychiatric inpatients.
New York State J Med. 1993; 16-17.

19. PHENYTOIN TO CONTROL THE AIDS!

After spending 17 years at Coler Hospital, I was to spend 15 years at MPC, in two installments. After the first four years at the latter, I left for an acute care teaching facility, Woodhull Hospital in northern Brooklyn, NY, hoping to further any of my studies, if I could. That was around 1992-3 and the scourge of the Acquired Immune Deficiency Syndrome (AIDS) was at its peak. It used to kill 95-100 persons a day in the U.S. alone.

These were young people, many in their teens and twenties. To keep the things in perspective, it should be noted that illnesses related to cigarette smoking killed 1350 people a day. The irony is, both of these are eminently preventable, not to mention obesity, with myself "pleading guilty as charged" to the last one.

There was no vaccine or another medical way to effectively prevent the AIDS. Newer medicines were coming out, but its control was still a remote goal, leave aside its cure. To see patients of their own age dying was too painful for the young interns and residents to bear. The "Only if" moment had been there for nearly fifteen years.

I had meticulously gone over Dryfus' book of references on phenytoin. There was a reference that claimed that phenytoin was effective in preventing the spread of the AIDS virus, at least in the *petri dish* in the lab. Later on I was to hear anecdotal reports from another neighboring teaching hospital that phenytoin was being used there for that very purpose. Prevention of the AIDS was not a well known application of phenytoin, nor was it approved by the FDA for that purpose. It deserved to be investigated.

The original report had come from none other than the discoverer of the AIDS virus, Montagnier from France. He had demonstrated that in the *tissue cultures*, when cells were grown in petri dishes, and if phenytoin was added to the cells before adding the *Human Immune-deficiency Virus* (HIV, which causes the AIDS), the cells could not be infected.

Similar results were obtained by adding serum from the healthy volunteers who had been given phenytoin orally before adding the virus. That means, even in therapeutic doses commonly used, and serum levels of phenytoin achieved on the wards, were effective in controlling the HIV infection. Note that *no virus was introduced in those volunteers*.

One question always bothers me, why even with such clear cut results and despite all facilities available to them, investigators do not do anything further? I had seen that with the team that had dripped calcium hydroxide in dialysis fluid to remove carbon dioxide and the membranes had clogged up. Why did they not try to isolate the reaction site with filters?

According to the Jain Indian philosophy of *Karmas*, this kind of talk is a disrespect to knowledge, and is punished by inability to succeed in one's pursuit of knowledge. A little soul searching can go a long way. Why was not I able to try peritoneal dialysis in patients? Also, why was not I able to give phenytoin to smokers to see whether it helped them quit and to lose weight? Research is an extremely fragile and precarious endeavor and limitations of previous researchers have to be appreciated, respected and overcome, rather than being judged unfairly.

With the help of a fully trained gastroenterologist awaiting his U.S credentials, Dr. Adnan Khdair (*Khu-dai-r*), I reviewed the medical records of patients who were receiving phenytoin and were tested to see whether they had the HIV infection and compared them with those who were tested for HIV but were not receiving phenytoin.

The results indicated that phenytoin therapy was associated with a lower likelihood of being infected with the HIV virus. In the data from Montagnier and others, it was shown that phenytoin prevented cells from filling up with calcium, an event that heralds the cell death. I took that to mean that phenytoin acts like a drug which blocks the calcium channels that lead from the surface to the interior of the cells.

Since I knew next to nothing of the cytopharmacology, my interpretation may or may not be valid, but it made me include, as a fallback strategy, patients who were receiving *calcium channel blocking drugs* like isradipine (Dynacirc, no longer marketed), amlodipine (Norvasc), etc., and found that some of these drugs were even more effective than phenytoin.

My paper was sent to a couple of journals and was rejected. No reason whatsoever was given. That was neither my first nor the last experience with my inability to kindle interest in the better knowledgeable others, even when we had nothing to offer to the AIDS patients. I have included that paper in the Part-II.

Possible use of phenytoin and of calcium channel blocking agents in controlling the HIV infection is still worth pursuing, especially for application in the under developed countries, if not in the developed ones. Let us draw a hypothesis.

***

Hypothesis:

1. Phenytoin has been found to be effective in preventing both, *primary* (virus entering a cell) and *secondary* (entering another cell after destroying one cell and coming out) *infections* of tissue cultures by the HIV virus.
2. Our data indicated that this is probably the case in human beings also.
3. Phenytoin apparently works as a calcium channel blocking agent.
4. Such agents like isradipine were found to be even more effective than phenytoin in preventing the HIV infection, that is patients receiving these drugs were less likely to be HIV positive.
5. Although dissimilar in many ways, all these patients were at perceived risk of HIV infection, as indicated by their being recommended for, and agreeing to be be tested for the HIV.
6. These drugs are not anti viral agents, but they protect the host cells themselves directly against the HIV. This is an unique mechanism of action.
7. These drugs are less toxic, and rather inexpensive compared to many anti viral drugs. There is no reason why they cannot be used together.

***

After the local petty politics made me earn my first pink slip (a layoff), I promptly moved to a nursing home in the Bronx. While there, I had a stroke caused by blood clots thrown to my brain from the neck vessels, requiring surgery to help me recover with practically no residual damage, except to entrench my delusion that whatever I was doing or trying to do in way of research was worthwhile.

I was trying to get the EKG and other papers published. I sent them to a prestigious journal, together with the illustrations. There were four such drawings that I have reproduced earlier in the chapter on EKG in this book. Their reviewers were absolutely unable to see anything that I was trying to show. For example, the legend said, "The P wave in this figure gets smaller with the forced water intake," the reviewers commented, "there is no P wave to be seen anywhere in that diagram."

The stroke had distorted my right-left perception (which I have recovered since). Therefore, when I arranged those figures #1-4 on the glass of the photocopy machine, I was looking at their back sides with labels indicating their figure numbers. On the front side which the reviewers saw was an entirely different arrangement. Well, that also happens.

While at the nursing home, I had an opportunity to deal with a nearby major medical center, to be on their staff and teach their residents. I obtained the meaningful membership (unlike what I had at the New York Medical College) of their medical board and had privileges to admit my patients there.

I shared my respiratory work with the Chairman of the Pulmonary Service there, who was an outstanding researcher of great reputation. Our ideas were complementary. He seemed to be interested in working with me. However, that was not going to be. I was laid off yet again before I could do anything along those lines. The project for which the nursing home had hired me was not getting off the ground, contrary to their lofty expectations.

Three more months after the stroke, I was laid off again within a six month period. Embattled, but not bitter, I went back to MPC.

20. BLOOD TRANSFUSION TO CURE HEPATITIS: B?

In the early 1990s my wife, Usha, was diagnosed to have Hepatitis: B infection, a viral disease, which was progressing to destroy her liver to make it fail. Four of her family members were to die of it by the end of that decade. There was nothing more I could do as a physician than to watch her go down the hill helplessly.

I did search the literature for any flimsy thing I could just grab on to sustain my hope. There was nothing. I called that Project: UB, combining the first initials of both of us. My by then 30 years old medical school picture of Hepatitis: B was that of an aggressive virus relentlessly attacking the liver and destroying it.

The literature told me that the picture was less violent, albeit, the outcome remained the same. The virus itself, related to the HIV causing the AIDS, is not *cytotoxic or* cells-destroying. Reaction of the body to fight it was responsible for much of the damage. Obviously, I was not going to prevent the body from defending itself by giving steroids and other drugs to curtail the fight.

Another problem was that the patients with Hepatitis: B of long standing continue to harbor the virus, but they produce no antibodies to fight it. Failure to fight is understandable, but failure to even initiate an opposition was strange.

I considered administering the Hepatitis: B vaccine that had become available recently, to stimulate the antibody production. Well, some workers had already tried it with the conclusion, it neither helps nor hurts. Anything that does not help can always hurt, even if we cannot see it.

There was yet another problem, a paper from the United Kingdom, in the New England Journal of Medicine reported. When someone is infected with the virus, it attaches itself onto the surface of that patient's *lymphocytes,* a kind of white blood cells. Lymphocytes in turn present the virus to the cells that can destroy the virus. There appeared to be some failure of this presenting mechanism.

I figured that maybe, that was the reason for absence of antibody response noted earlier. However, there were many other patients who had been vaccinated and who had produced the antibodies to the virus. These antibodies were capable of clearing the virus from the body.

My response as a Letter to the Editor was delayed and rejected. I have presented it in Part-II of this book. In Usha's family, more on her mother's side, several people had died of fulminant Hepatitis: B. Even though, mother to children transmission at the time of delivery has been postulated, it has been not adequately explained. I am not going to address that either.

Why can we not administer *antibodies* or the whole blood? We can settle for plasma, the liquid part of the blood without the cells, but containing the antibody proteins. We can use the HepBig (Hepatitis: B Immune Globulin) infusion. There are better drugs coming up on the market, and we may not need to resort to this any longer.

Usha deteriorated too rapidly for me to think this through and try it out. Such studies take months to design, set up and execute. However, she did receive blood transfusions[18] to correct her severe anemia in 1993 and she did get better.

Whether that was due to the general tonic effect of blood or a specific one on the virus, I do not know. Nor do I know whether that blood contained any antibodies to the Hepatitis: B virus. Soon her case became too serious for amateur research and too unsettling for me to think it through.

After her transplant[19] in 1999, she did receive every other month, the Hepatitis: B immune globulin, HepBig which carries the antibodies, along with other antiviral drugs and steroids to suppress the body's reaction—not to the virus, that I was referring to, but to prevent the body from rejecting the transplanted organ.

Hypothesis:

Usha's family members succumbed to a very aggressive and stormy disease. There may be some genetic predisposition for this violent form of the disease, even though no genetic link is suspected for the vertical transmission of the disease.

---

[18]   A family with HBV and hepatic decompensation. In
       Questions, Answers, and Exclamations:
       From the Garage of a Clinical Researcher. P. 281-82, 2011.
       Setubandh Publications, New York.

[19]   More than twelve years after the transplant, she is doing well. I have chronicled our journey through the transplant experience in a documentary novel, *Dawn at Midnight* (*Sameepe* in Gujarati). Please see the end pages for more information.

21. CAN'T WE ALL BE
SOMEWHAT IMMUNO-SUPPRESSED?

There is nothing silly about a new idea. Like newborn babies, they all may look strange and unlike anything else. We used to get sick with diarrhea and sore throat when we visited India. We still do and rather more so with our increasing age. However, I have noticed that my wife Usha, after her liver transplant is getting sick less often and when she does get sick, it is less severe than the rest of us.

She is on prednisone and tacrolimus (Prograf) in minimal doses. She was warned about immunosuppression making her more vulnerable to the usual and the unusual infections. The warning should have been better given to us. My feeling is, immunosuppression of a lower magnitude may do all of us some good.

This may look like an overkill, not if you have ever ruined your vacation or a part of it, fighting those travelers' travails!

✱✱✱

EYES, ENT, AND GENERAL SURGERY

22 (A). WOUND HEALING GOES UP IN SMOKE!

After a hiatus of six years I returned to MPC having given up all hopes of furthering my work and collecting two layoffs and a stroke to show as profit. After a brief stint as the Chief of Medical Services, I had returned to the direct patient care and had good respect and support from the newly hired chief, Dr. Rogelio Foster. He used to consult me and others in the department. For complicated projects requiring some statistical or other special analysis, either I volunteered for or he assigned them to me.

One problem of great importance and imminence that confronted us was that of failure of our patients to heal after surgeries done at another hospital. Many of our patients developed major complications, delaying the wound healing which kept them away from their psychiatric therapy.

MPC had limited facility to provide more than minimal postoperative care, despite its devoted nursing staff. Keeping the patients at the other hospital was expensive. At times we had to send our staff to be with our patients there. That was not cost effective.

In a couple of meetings with their administration and with their surgical chief, nothing concrete came about. The chief of surgery contended that his results were very good and blamed the non-healing wounds on our ineptness. Even if we accepted his argument, still we were at a loss to explain what was happening.

1. What we were seeing was the large abdominal *wounds opening up completely* (called *dehiscence*), often exposing the internal organs. This is generally a life threatening complication, killing more than 50% of the victims. Fortunately its occurrence was said to be very rare, except in our patients, none of whom fortunately died.

2. *Repeat surgery* was required more often to remove the huge collections of liters of fluid from around the surgical wounds. Such water swellings are called *Seroma*, or a collection of blood serum. Some patients required repeated aspirations of their seroma.

3. *Weakening of the abdominal wall at the site of the incision*, with internal elements trying to push out, called an *incisional hernia*, was also common.

These complications occurred with various kinds of operations and there was no definite pattern to them. I volunteered my services to investigate the situation. I had no idea what I was to find and how. It was a fishing expedition.

Besides being a curious person and having done some research work, I was trained in running the medical audits to solve day to day problems, e.g., patients falling down in certain wards, medical records remaining uncompleted, etc. This kind of work demands forgetting all assumed causes and doing a thorough analysis of meticulously gathered voluminous data.

There are known factors that affect healing of surgical wounds. These include diabetes, poor nutrition, low protein level, vitamin deficiency, immune suppression, cancers, steroid therapy and so on.

Working with Dr. Foster, I collected the names of all patients who had any kind of surgery within the past 18 months, with at least a one inch long visible wound. Then I gathered data on above mentioned and other such factors that can impair healing. I also retrieved general information like blood count, height, weight, smoking habit, drug abuse, diagnosis of the AIDS and anything else that caught my eye.

For each of these factors, I ran a comparison between those who had a delayed wound healing and those whose postoperative course was uneventful. Since physicians generally correct the known causes of delayed healing, none of the latter were found to differ between the groups. The only variable that stood out as being different was their smoking habits.

All patients with the post operative complications turned out to be heavy smokers, despite hospital's policy against uncontrolled smoking. They smoked more cigarettes (their own) per day, demanded to smoke between the scheduled cigarette breaks and became agitated when their demands were not met.

The control group with uncomplicated post operative course was found to contain nonsmokers or minimal smokers, that is, who smoked fewer than permitted number of cigarettes, sometimes skipping them altogether, they never asked for more cigarettes, did not demand to smoke between the scheduled time and never got agitated when their request was denied. Even though smoking is generally known to impair wound healing, there are very few reports of smoking related impaired wound healing in living patients as opposed to lab animals.

***

22 (B). SMOKE AND MIRRORS OF SCIENCE

There was another interesting finding. Patients born during certain months of the year were more likely to have a complicated course. This association was statistically even stronger than that with cigarette smoking. No other factor studied shared this association with the month of birth.

In psychiatric literature, there are reports of Schizophrenia and other diseases being associated with certain calendar months in which the patient was born. There are medical conditions also, in which such findings are reported. Some of these are contradictory, especially when data from both, the southern and the northern hemispheres are pooled. No such claims have been put forward in case of wound healing.

What could possibly be the importance of such esoteric and academically strange relationship? In research, most often you start with a question and try to find an answer. However, there are times when you are faced with an answer and are called upon to find the question, akin to the TV game show "Jeopardy."

Many diseases are caused by genetic factors. Many more are probably caused indirectly by making one genetically vulnerable. There may be influence of viral and other diseases occurring in pregnant mothers that can affect a child. These are not clearly understood and they never will be if we decide to ignore them altogether.

To clarify, we are not talking about whether the operation was done in January or in July. We are talking about the month of birth, for which no surgeon is going to be blamed. Back home in India, during my childhood and even later on, I had heard my mother and others talk about[20] "pro-septic body" of some children whose abrasions and cuts were more likely to get infected, whereas in others they healed well.

Maybe, that vulnerability is associated with being born during a certain time of the year. One does not have to believe in astrology to understand and appreciate this. I submitted the paper to a few psychiatric journals, hoping that it would interest them and help their readers address the issue of inpatient smoking in a new light. It did not.

I sent it to a leading surgical journal. It apparently liked the paper but, one of its reviewers called the association with the month of birth "bizarre," with understandable reasoning and asked me to revise the paper, deleting everything about the month of birth. I was interested in truth and scientific inquiry, rather than just getting published and thereby fostering the notions that have not been challenged with a scientific scrutiny.

Why was my insistence on such a strange and unknown finding? It is not relevant whether I believed in it or not. I do not know anything more than anybody else about it. My refusal to drop that reference to the month of birth was precisely because it is strange, unknown and yes, bizarre. In research, that is called *terra incognita* or the unknown territory. If we are to deny its existence, we might as well lock up the house of science!

Psychiatric journals found the observations to be only of interest to surgeons and the latter would not have anything to do with anything softer than concrete. I believed, and still do, that it was concrete.

---

[20] It is called "પાકણી માટી" in Gujarati. Earth or soil is one of the five elements that the body is made of. Literally, it says, *Septic Soil*.

23. THE NOSE WITH A SPLIT PERSONALITY

Before we leave the cigarette smoking and pulmonary respiration, I should mention in passing a couple of ideas that I had toyed with.

A. Replacing a Tracheostomy Tube

This is the "L" shaped tube that is placed in the trachea through a surgically made hole in front of the neck. That tube can be connected to a ventilator, or may be kept just to remove the secretions using a suction cannula to protect the patient from *asphyxiation* or choking. This tube needs to be replaced with a new one every few days or weeks.

The tube gets very stiff and its surface gets rough with dried up secretions inside and around it, making it difficult for the doctor changing it, and painful for the patient. Removing the tube is generally not very difficult. Inserting a clean tube through ever narrowing, inflamed and fragile passages gets progressively tougher and tougher.

In medicine, to affix a needle on to a syringe without threads or a lock to hold the needle in place, it is customary to put the needle on and turning it half a turn as if tightening a screw while pressing it. This *half turn technique* was applied by me to replacing the tracheostomy tube making my life and that of the patient easier.

The problem is, the tube is angled, rather than being straight like a syringe and needle pair. Once inserted successfully, its shorter arm points straight out and the longer one rests in the trachea pointing downwards. Trying to push it in first and then down is difficult as described.

Turning it by half turn while inserting it, makes the shorter arm point upwards making it impossible to push the inner end down. I tried starting the "wrong way" with the shorter arm pointing up and the other one straight through the hole. While pushing the tube inside and swiftly downwards, its shorter end is twisted for half a turn, like the handle of a money safe, to make the insertion successful.

I have had tried this method innumerable times and it was received well by my patients. Many have had preferred to wait for my return from a short vacation or a weekend to get their tube replaced on a non-emergency basis.

This method was published[21] in the Residents and Staff Physicians in the 1970s. I was paid $15 for that. That was the only money I was to receive for my research related work, I think.

B. Why Do Patients with a Tracheostomy Like to Have It Suctioned?

When the upper airways are full of secretions, patients cannot breathe and if they have a tracheostomy, they cannot cough the sticky secretions out. Removing these secretions using a suction machine understandably makes them feel relived.

I had noticed that many a time, a patient sitting in a chair, or resting comfortably in bed, with no apparent need for suctioning, called the staff nurse, to do the suctioning through his tracheostomy tube. The patient appreciated it when the nurse obliged either right away or a little later.

---

[21]   Replacing a tracheostomy tube.
Resident and Staff Physician. 1974. 64:318.

I have thought about it for a long time. What possible benefit can a patient get from that apparently superfluous suctioning? I have heard the usual explanations like dependence, attention seeking behavior, anxiety and so on. All these may of course be there but, as I have had always done, I liked to probe deeper for the real reason.

Hypothesis:
1. We do know that tracheal suctioning is potentially a life threatening procedure. We are taking the patient from the sea level to the top of the Mt. Everest within seconds by rapidly lowering the pressure in the upper airways. That can cause severe lack of oxygen or *hypoxemia* and maybe, death.
2. In patients with a tracheostomy and ventilator therapy, when resting without the ventilator, and often without the oxygen administration, carbon dioxide level in their blood and in the air sacs in their lungs increases and correspondingly the oxygen level decreases.
3. The mechanism of shortness of breath or *dyspnoea* which occurs with low oxygen level is not quite clear, but the latter stimulates breathing efforts uncomfortable to the patient unable to execute them because of stiff lungs.
4. These patients with *emphysema* or air trapping are unable to breathe in because their lungs are, as it is, full of trapped air. They can choke on air, literally. The real problem in emphysema patients is not as much with breathing in, as it is with breathing out, or rather not breathing out. The patient is unable to breathe in without expelling the trapped air first. Breathing in deeply, worsens the air trapping.

5. Their attempts to force the air out makes the airways collapse prematurely, by squeezing everything.
6. Suctioning does not squeeze the airways, even though it does increase the difference between the pressure around and that within the airways. This needs to be verified.
7. Suctioning can remove the choking caused by the trapped air, can remove the trapped air by creating a negative pressure, can remove some carbon dioxide and thereby permit the oxygen level to increase, without itself giving any oxygen per se.
8. In essence, *suctioning may be acting as a negative pressure ventilator*, not in the usual sense of the term which refers to respirators like the iron lungs, sucking the air in by creating a negative pressure in and around the chest, but rather by sucking the air out, that is, *inducing an active expiration.*
9. This may be an artificial way of achieving the *corporeal,* or by the body itself, removal of carbon dioxide, as opposed to the extracorporeal one via the ECMO and a far less *traumatic,* that is, injurious one at that.
10. This may be a more sensible way, in contrast to the positive-pressure, volume-cycled respirators that brutally push the air in, or the negative pressure ventilators which are not effective in decreasing the air trapping.
11. This property of suctioning needs further exploring for its potential for becoming a life sustaining innovative procedure.
12. Compressed air or oxygen can be administered simultaneously.
13. This may offer another modality of treatment, besides modified peritoneal dialysis.

I have had not done any actual work on this as such, except to work on the Hemorespirators and the dialysis project to think through these principles. This may be the simplest way to achieve the salvation. It is said, "The truth is simple!" This is our chance to see that for ourselves.

C. The Nose with a Split Personality:

God or whatever else you believe in, has given us two eyes, two ears, two breasts, but only one heart and one nose, or so we are led to believe. There are two sides of the heart, right and left, with four chambers. Our nose has two distinct orifices or openings, leading into two cavities separated by the *septum* or a partition. Nature has not done so with our tongue. Why with the nose?

We rarely pay attention to our noses long enough to notice that both "noses" (*nostrils* refers to the entrance openings only) breathe independently. At any moment we may be breathing through one, or the other, or through both of them. They keep on alternating their duties, switching over several times a day, on their own.

During my high school years I had read in one of our Jain religious books about the *sun breath* and the *moon breath*, that is breathing happening through the right or the left side of the nose. The book then went on to list all the good and bad things that can be predicted based on which side is found to work at a particular time, including say, death can occur if a sun breath did not occur for a few hours on the new year. There were also predictions of the sex of the child to be conceived that night based on the kind of breath.

Most of the above predictions cannot be put as a scientific question as defined by Popper, that is in a form in which it can be disproved. Faithful believers may try it out. I could not find much in the medical literature about these respiratory cycles, in the 1970s when I decided to look into the matter.

There were reports confirming their existence and that they were affected by body position and by drugs like *adrenaline* that cause blood vessels to shrink. The dependent side of the nose receives more blood and its passages thus swollen, limit the airflow through that side, while the other one opens up.

Changing one's position from lying on one side to the other can close one side and open the other. The sun or moon breath can also be affected by applying adrenaline which shrinks the local blood vessels to open up the passage on that side.

I wanted to investigate this, but had no grant money for it. Talking to my colleague in the neurology department of Coler Hospital revealed that they had an EEG (brain waves) machine which was equipped to record nasal breathing simultaneously. He ordered two electrodes for me, since they had never used that function of the machine. I was able to record the differential breathing of both sides, but there was no definite hypothesis to pursue.

This is a less crowded field for those who want to pursue it. However there must be a reason why it is not more crowded. Any assumptions one makes may be at one's own risk.

★★★

24. WATCHING THE SUGAR WITH THE EYES AND VICE VERSA[22]

Long term effects of diabetes mellitus on the eyes are well known. Diabetes can cause cataracts and vascular changes in the retina, resulting in diminished vision and blindness. In the shorter run, it can affect refraction and change the strength of the glasses needed. Optometrists prefer to do the *refraction* when a diabetic patient's blood sugar is within the normal range and is stable.

Once my own newly made glasses were found to be useless in a week or so. The correction provided was off by a power of two *diopters* (the so called "numbers" like +2 or -3.5). My blood sugar was found to be out of range and out of control.

The above is quite well known. However, the day to day change in blood sugar and its effect on refraction are not well appreciated, although it is supposedly well known. The lens in our eye absorbs glucose and depending upon the concentration of the latter, it either swells by absorbing water, or shrinks by losing some. Either of these affects the power of the lens.

If the changes in the thickness of the lens are sensitive and reproducible enough, there is a possibility that we can substitute the vision test for the more painful finger stick blood glucose determination and thereby improve patient's compliance with testing the sugar. Finger

---

[22] *Citation:*   Shah BS
Watching the sugar with the eyes, and vice versa, in
Questions, Answers, and Exclamations
From the Garage of a Clinical Researcher, p.141-145,
Setubandh Publications, New York. 2011.

stick test is far more sensitive and objective, but the vision test is likely to be more acceptable.

I used the *Rosenbaum's chart for reading test* to check my own vision and did a finger stick glucose just after it. I did this for several days and plotted a scatter diagram shown in figure: 8.

The horizontal axis shows daily blood sugar readings. The vertical axis shows the *denominator* (the bottom number) from the vision 20/40, 20/60, etc. The higher the number, the worse the vision. Similarly, the higher the sugar level, the worse it is.

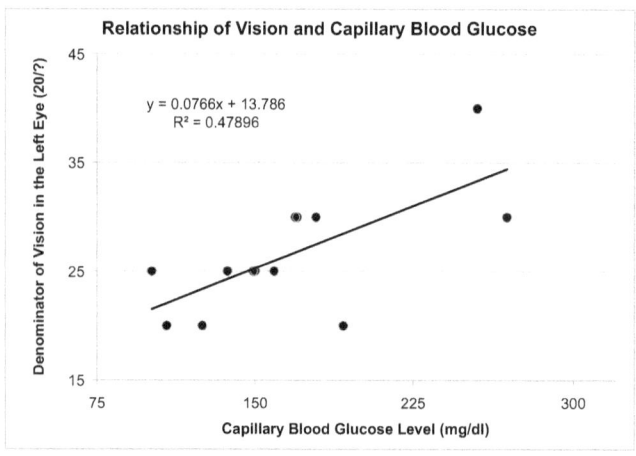

Figure: 8 shows relation between blood sugar and vision. For example, when sugar is 125 mg/dl the vision is 20/20, see the bottom row middle point. When the sugar is 250, the vision is 20/40 (the highest data point).

The above relationship is statistically significant at 2% level, or $p < 0.02$. That is good enough. However, there is a technical glitch here. Sugar and vision both are measured at certain interval on a time line. Therefore these data constitute what is called a *time series* and a different kind of statistical approach is required to be acceptable.

Instead of taking the values of both variable at a certain time, we calculate how much they have changed over the preceding interval, a day in our data. This change is represented with a triangular symbol, the Greek letter Δ, known as *Delta*. "ΔSugar" means change in sugar and "Δvision" indicates that in vision.

In the following figure: 9, I have plotted Δsugar against Δvision. The graph still shows the same relationship, but the association is closer and stronger. The relationship is significant at 1% level, p < 0.01. The line drawn on the graph is called the *regression line* which describes the relationship between the two variables.

When the blood sugar increases, the vision worsens, the record moves downwards and to our right along the line. When sugar decreases, the vision improves and the record moves upwards and to our left. This is called an *inverse, negative*, or *reciprocal* relationship.

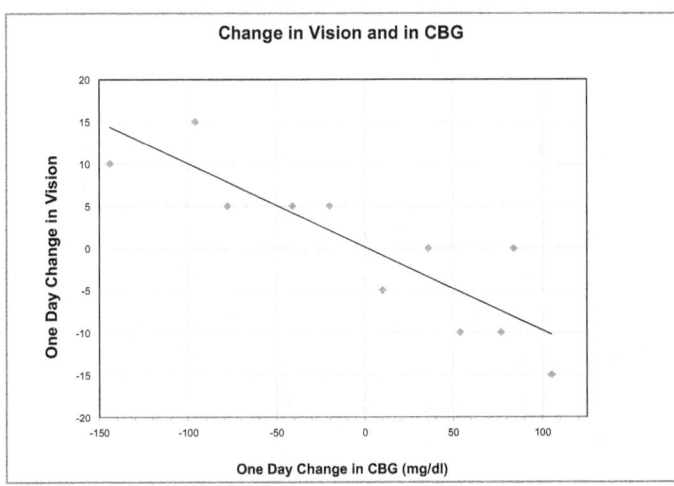

Figure: 9. Change in sugar and that in vision over the last one day are plotted against each other. These results are highly significant, p < 0.01. CBG means capillary blood glucose or finger stick sugar.

If there is a cataract in one eye, that eye cannot be used for this purpose. Fortunately the vision in the other eye would serve the same purpose. This plot has to be generated for that particular patient. A plot generated for one patient cannot be used as such for another one.

The plot in figure: 9 represents data gathered from myself. Now, let us say that my vision was 20/20 yesterday and the corresponding blood sugar was 150 mg/dl. If the vision is 20/35 today, that is a worsening change of 15, (that is, minus 15 in the denominator), my projected sugar is expected to be higher by 100 mg/dl (the lower end of the line), or it is expected to be 250 mg/dl.

Changes in the sugar in the optic lens disturbs the water balance within the lens. A high concentration of sugar makes the lens absorb more water from its surroundings and consequently the lens swells. That in turn affects the thickness of the lens and its optic power. These changes take some time to occur. Probably therefore, our results showing the change over the last 24 hours (figure: 9) were better than the simultaneous ones (figure: 8).

***

If for any reason, the lens has become inelastic, unable to swell and shrink with changes in blood glucose and those in its water content, the vision may not change. My right eye has had a stable cataract, and that eye did not show any change in its visual acuity with that in blood glucose. Figures: 8 and 9 show the data for my left eye.

About a year after the above work was done, I found that neither of my eyes reflected changes in my blood sugar level. The vision always remained stable at 20/20. This needs to be investigated. My suspicion is, maybe, I am developing a cataract in my left eye as well. The cataract may not even be visible yet. That is interesting, because the inelasticity of the lens is becoming apparent even before the cataract can be seen.

Hypothesis:
1. Visual acuity of eyes faithfully reflect the systemic changes in the blood sugar level, in absence of cataract, etc.
2. In a given individual, this finding can enable us to monitor blood glucose in a painless and hence more acceptable manner.
3. Failure of an eye to reflect the changes in blood sugar by those in the vision may indicate an inelastic lens and it may herald the beginning of a cataract.
4. Inelasticity of the optic lens with a developing cataract may become apparent on the vision chart, even before the cataract is visible.

This method needs more work and it has to be standardized to make it more practical. A submission of a letter to the editor about this was rejected, and it has *not* been reproduced in part: II either.

PSYCHIATRIC DISORDERS

25. PANIC DISORDER
DEPRESSION and SUICIDE

Doctors learn from their patients' diseases and afflictions. However, the best way to learn about any disease is to have it. Nothing provides one a better opportunity to observe a disease subjectively and objectively than that. It also effectively serves as a role reversal for a doctor to be in patients' shoes.

With that in mind, I had the good fortune of suffering from panic disorder[23]. It manifests itself as a series of severe *anxiety attacks, without any discernible reason* for the anxiety, unlike the usual panic that comes with facing an audience, one's boss, first date, or an exam for which one is not prepared at all.

Panic disorder can and does mimic heart attack, stomach problem and many other conditions; to make it more complicated, it can coexist with them. Making its diagnosis may be delayed for many years, but its treatment is generally not difficult.

Patient may have many associated *phobias* or fears, like that of height, crowded places, open places, closed ones like elevators, highway ramps, swimming pools and so on. Many patients being afraid of driving give up their jobs, lock themselves in their room, get depressed and may even commit suicide.

------

[23] See "My life with panic disorder" in the list of books on the last page.

There are many potential research ideas about panic disorder and related conditions, that I have raised in the book on panic disorder. I will only enumerate them here:

1. Is panic disorder caused by the mind divided between what one is called upon to do vis a vis what one would rather do? Therapists have lamented, *only if the patients would be more assertive!* Maybe, there is a reason why they are not and it is causing the conflict.

2. Can it be induced by drinking guava juice? Or, does the latter mimic a panic attack by lowering the blood glucose?

3. Does it have anything to do with being in a shoe store, especially that in Ahmedabad, India. I had several attacks while in the shoe stores there, but never in the U.S.

4. Can drugs like glucophage (Metformin) and others used to treat diabetes, induce suicidal ideations in patients with panic disorder? I had such experience with glucophage and two other drugs. The evidence against them was circumstantial and not conclusive. I have prescribed these drugs to psychiatric patients without any untoward effect. However, this needs to be explored.

5. How can a patient with panic disorder have a feeling of loneliness when he denies it vehemently? Such feeling disappears when the attack subsides. A lonely feeling is not expected to vanish in a few minutes. I used to walk away from the company I loved, during the attacks.

6. Similarly, how can a patient have suicidal ideations, while insisting that he dreads the idea of killing himself? I used to call such thoughts *suicidal intrusions*, because I positively and categorically did not want to kill myself.

7. The loneliness-depression-suicide cycle is known quite well and it maybe valid, however, I think that these can occur in a different sequence, that is, suicidal intrusions that the patient disavows, can put him in a battle against death in which nobody can help him, thereby engendering a feeling of helplessness and loneliness which can lead to depression.

I would reproduce in the Part: II, a couple of articles that I wrote during June 2004, for thinking through while I was right in the middle of suffering from suicidal ideations. It can be interesting for a general reader but it is a bit too long for this part and is better suited for a researcher.

26. VIOLENCE IN PSYCHIATRIC INPATIENTS

From the self directed violence like suicide, let us now turn to that directed at other patients, staff members, property, furniture, glass windows, etc. Such violence includes verbal and physical agitation, threatening, abuse, assault with or without a weapon, and rape, among other things.

Inpatient violence includes homicides and suicide which unfortunately do happen in the mental health facilities, but luckily in numbers too small to be subjected to a statistical analysis. Violence is expensive, not only because of pain and suffering, but also because of the trauma to the staff who has to control it, has to accompany the violent patient for care of cuts, wound and fractures to an acute care hospital.

Violence makes other patients nervous, destroys the harmony of a team, makes the perpetrator feel guilty and there are legal issues. Discharging a violent patient to the community or a custodial care facility or a foster family is extremely time consuming, generally frustrating and futile.

When I joined MPC, part of my assignment was to provide medical care to the severely violent patients in the Intensive Psychiatric Service (IPS), equivalent to an ICU. I was not experienced in dealing with them. Therefore two ward psychiatrists and other staff stood guard for any possible contingencies, when I was with a patient who had just been involved in an altercation.

MPC was on the forefront of research on violence and there was a study in progress to do video monitoring for unappreciated or unreported violence and factors leading up to it.

I am from a vegetarian family, practicing an extremely nonviolent religion Jainism which tries to protect even the invisible life in the air and in the water. I had never had killed a rat or a roach or an ant. I have no idea how I got interested in studying violence.

Probably my long standing habit of going to the root of any unsolved problem was behind it. The psychiatric literature is full of violence of inpatients and of the prison inmates and criminals at large. My interest was in looking for medical factors that can lead to violence or help predicting it.

There are diseases and conditions like *epilepsy, hyperthyroidism, hypoglycemia* (low blood sugar), head trauma, which can be associated with violent behavior. Drug abuse, alcoholism and some psychiatric conditions like *paranoia* (over-suspiciousness) can also lead to violence. These are well known for their effect on behavior.

What I was looking for was something in the patients' history, a laboratory test result, any drug therapy, that was associated with violence, without necessarily causing it. Such marker can tell us in advance to forestall the violent event. The lab test had to be common enough to be generally performed routinely in almost all patients on admission, to have any predictor value.

Low level of blood cholesterol had been reported to be such an indicator. Most of the studies were *retrospective* chart reviews which are done after the fact. Even then the results were equivocal and had generated some controversy. Arguments tend to get confusing, when people argue about different aspects of an issue simultaneously. Some investigators disputed the findings, while others were opposed to stopping the cholesterol lowering therapy to thwart violence and thereby risk increasing the likelihood of a heart attack.

Most of the studies in the literature had looked at the level of the total cholesterol including its fractions, namely, the good *(HDL, High Density Lipoprotein)* cholesterol, the bad *(LDL, Low Density Lipoprotein)* cholesterol, plus the fatty particles *(Triglycerides)*.

With increasing prevalence of obesity nationwide and more so in psychiatric patients being treated with modern *atypical psychotropic drugs* and in those being treated for the AIDS, it had become a standard practice to do these tests of cholesterol levels, collectively known as *lipid panels or lipid profiles* on admission in all patients.

Our study entailed retrieving the names of the patients involved in assaultive behavior. These were always recorded on a special event report. The data showed that the patients involved in a violent assault, either as the attacker or as a victim *both* had abnormal *cholesterol fractions* on admission. Victims and attacker both came from the same population and often their roles were interchangeable.

It was easy to see the reason for the controversy surrounding the role of total cholesterol. The total cholesterol was indeed a poor predictor of violence. In my data, it was the HDL or the *good cholesterol* fraction that was decreased and the LDL or the *bad cholesterol* was increased.

There was no reason at all for not lowering the level of the LDL in violent patients, just as in those who were not violent. It has always been recommended for protection of the heart and the coronary arteries. Similarly, for all patients it was considered desirable to have a relatively higher HDL cholesterol.

Many controversies would subside if we first define exactly what it is that we are fighting about. The data showed that the decreased total cholesterol is not always associated with a violent tendency. The two fractions that were associated with violence were candidates to be treated regardless of violence. What was good for the heart was also good for the brain.

To recapitulate:
1. Total cholesterol level is a poor predictor of violence.
2. A high level of LDL cholesterol (the *bad* one) showed a tendency for being associated with future violence.
3. A low level of HDL (good) cholesterol showed a statistically significant inverse association with a future violent event.
4. The current standards for correcting any of the above for the cardiac prevention can be safely applied to prevention of violence as well, there being no reason for a controversy.

The full paper[24] on this topic is included in the Part: II. The paper was rejected by medical and psychiatric journals.

---

24 Revisiting the cholesterol-violence controversy with new observations on various lipid fractions: A retrospective study. In Questions, Answers, and Exclamations from the Garage of a Clinical Researcher. P. 229 - 243, 2011 Setubandh Publications, New York.

27. BIRDS OF THE SAME FEATHERS?

Having failed in getting anybody interested in my reconciling the opposite sides of the controversy over lowering the cholesterol level in violent patients, by demonstrating their congruence, I turned my attention to see whether various psychiatric patients differed in their lipid profile or analysis of cholesterols.

We generally hear about cholesterol only in a negative context, whenever something goes wrong. That makes one forget that it is an essential substance in our body for manufacturing the sex hormones and those to fight stress. Both these affect our behavior and therefore, it makes sense to see whether various behaviors are associated with different patterns of cholesterol.

There were several distinct groups of patients characterized by various degrees of *going against the doctors' advice*. These groups were,

1. Assaultive, aggressive patients, and their victims
2. Diabetic patients requiring admission to a special ward
3. Resistant Smokers
4. Drug abusers
5. *Polydipsia* patients with uncontrolled water drinking
6. Sexual predators
7. Control group with none of the above.

I should have included in the above, the maverick research workers going against everything that we know to be true, trying to prove it wrong and thereby breaking all the rules of the norm. I could not find enough of them to run a statistical analysis.

This entire topic requires in depth knowledge and firsthand experience with providing medical care, to understand and appreciate the significance of the findings of this study. This paper is presented[25] in its entirety in the Part: II.

---

[25] Lipid profile of various groups of nonconforming psychiatric inpatients. In Questions, Answers, and Exclamations from the Garage of a Clinical Researcher. P. 244 - 254, 2011 Setubandh Publications, New York.

28. TAMING THE BEAST
MAKING THE CLOZARIL TREATMENT SAFER

Clozaril (Clozapine) is a newer drug of the class known as the *atypical psychotropics*. It is a very powerful and effective drug for severe resistant *psychosis, schizophrenia*, violence and suicide. Unfortunately it is highly toxic. It was withdrawn initially because it was found to lower the white blood cells count precariously.

It was reintroduced with the proviso that weekly monitoring of the white blood cells (called *WBC, Leucocytes, Neutrophils*). It has many other major side effects, e.g., anemia, severe constipation, seizures, weakness and drop spells. Many of these require the patient to be referred to an acute care hospital. This has had prevented many patients from benefitting from this drug.

My self imposed mission was to come up with a strategy to predict and prevent the complications associated with clozaril treatment. This turned out to be a fascinating study. It is a shame that a very useful and effective drug cannot be administered to many who need it the most, in adequate doses. My boss Dr. Foster worked with me on this.

The data showed a relatively simple and clinically applicable way to predict and possibly prevent severe complications of clozapine therapy. I could not generate any interest from either medical or psychiatric journals in the full paper. This paper is produced[26] in its entirety in Part: II.

✶✶✶

---

26 Risk factors for acute medical complications associated with clozapine treatment: A retrospective study. In
Questions, Answers, and Exclamations from the
Garage of a Clinical Researcher. P. 256 - 271, 2011
Setubandh Publications, New York.

IT'S NOT OVER YET!

29. WORKING WITH THE ARTIFICIAL BRAIN!

Like someone else's dreams, someone else's ideas are not ours. No, I am not having second thoughts about publishing my ideas. What I am referring to is the motivation, intense interest, determination, addictive attachment and a strong nurturing instinct that go in taking the ideas to fruition.

It is in our hand to control what enters our minds. Once an idea enters, or *infects* our minds, the former has a will of its own. New ideas are frightening and most of us would rather remain miles away from them. This chapter is for those who would rather jump into the oncoming waves instead.

One has to know the laws to break them. One cannot question a law without knowing what it is. Something has to cease making sense to us, before we pay attention to it. The realization that there is no Santa Claus, nor is there a tooth ferry distinct from one's father or mother, can leave one in an insipid world.

Those fantasies have to be substituted for by newer ones, more tantalizing, more inviting and more powerful. These come from observing the nature and everything around us. Someone has said, "Paradox is the truth standing on its head just to draw our attention." Let me present a few that I have come across:

A. It is Twenty-three, Dummy!

Once my wife and I were going over our household expenses, during the early days of our marriage, when our son was maybe, two or three years old. My wife started adding up the numbers to come to a halt at, "Fifteen plus eight comes to,…comes to….," when we heard, "Twenty-three." Both of us looked at each other in disbelief, as neither of us had said that.

We looked at our son playing next to us. He was the only one who could have said that and there was no doubt that he had. He did not know what *twenty-three* meant. The TV or the radio was not on either. What are the odds of his coming out with that *answer*? Maybe, our son was going to be a precocious child with some kind of gift.

That was 35 years or so ago and our son has turned out to be a bright young man, to become an attending physician at a prestigious medical center, but apart from that he has not turned out to be any different. We are still waiting though. What can we make of it? Both of us were hallucinating? Without taking any drugs? Well, we may never know, or someday, maybe we will!

B. You Can't See Him, He is Dead!

We were making our daily ward rounds on the respiratory ward of the V. A. Hospital during my fellowship, with the senior attending, walking and stopping in the long corridor often. We wanted all patients to be in their rooms in their beds, so that we would not miss anybody.

There was an old man with dementia. I remember his name, a Mr. Brady, who was in the habit of pacing the same hallway. He ignored our requests to return to his room halfway down the hall. He wanted to know, "Why?"

We explained to him, but he insisted that we could see him right there and that there was nothing else that we were going to do, which was not quite untrue. Then we told him that he was in our way and that we wanted to finish the rounds.

"You want to see everybody?" He asked.

"Yes." We replied.

"Even the guy in the last room?" There were four patients in that last room. We answered affirmatively.

"You can't see him. He died last night." He mumbled. We looked at the nurse, who confirmed that she had seen all four patients alive that morning. It was already past ten o'clock. None of the patients was particularly sick either.

When we reached the last room at our regular pace, maybe, after 15-20 minutes, three patients were sitting up or were lying down and reading. No curtains were drawn. The fourth patient was indeed, dead!

To date I have not been able to make any sense out of it. Coincidence, chance, fluke, even truth, all were considered by us and then by me repeatedly over the years. It just does not make sense.

C. Cars are Human, too!

Cars are, well, as human as their drivers are. Animated films may leave with you with an erroneous impression that cars need to be animated. The truth is otherwise. In an earlier chapter (EKG Waves) in this book I gave you an example of my car responding to my angry determination and getting to roll again.

We had two Hondas of different years, and then we had two Toyotas of different model years. When I replaced the battery on one, I had to do that for the other, too. It did not matter whether one had almost one and half time as many miles as the jealous one.

We had decided to send one to the salvage yard after having it through almost two hundred thousand miles. A friend of ours insisted on taking it against our advice. It stayed in the friend's driveway for one year or more, when its younger sister broke the axle. Both were donated to a charity simultaneously.

Elevators, lawn movers, computers, and other machines have a mind of their own, and probably a heart with feelings as well. Someday, we will be able to understand one another.

D. Is There Death Before Life?

At Coler Hospital, when I was in charge of the respiratory rehabilitation unit, a young girl with respiratory failure and a tracheostomy was admitted. She used to be visited and was generally surrounded by many young and strange looking friends.

One morning she went into cardiorespiratory arrest. Resuscitation was done by an entire team of doctors, nurses, respiratory therapists, etc. It was not difficult to assist her breathing, since she already had the tracheostomy in place. She was given oxygen.

Her heart soon showed a straight line on the EKG and we could not hear any heart beats either. She was a relatively slim woman, without any emphysema which can obscure the heart sounds.

After half an hour of unsuccessful CPR, she was declared dead and the team departed, leaving me to fill out the death certificate, inform the family, etc. The head nurse started cleaning up the mess.

"Dr. Shah!" I heard the nurse call me in near panic. I looked at her and did not take long to figure out, why. The patient was moving her limbs on her own! We just stood there. The patient returned to her usual self within a couple of hours, to die after two more weeks.

Illicit drugs is one possibility. She was not visited by anyone that morning. She may have had some in her possession. Drugs appear to be the obvious explanation. Drug screens were not done commonly then. Maybe, we do know the answer in this case, or do we? I am not sure.

There are many such events and anecdotes waiting for someone to come along and explain. The reader may be able to add a few more of his or her own, and may be able to recall many from the magazines and other media.

E. One's Own Problem!

With due respect to Alexander Pope who said *Little knowledge is a dangerous thing*, I think that ignorance disguised as knowledge is the worst.

Medicine also shrouds its ignorance under euphemistic terminology. We tell a patient with some skin rash that (s)he has *dermatosis*, which essentially means a *skin condition*. We are telling the patient exactly the same thing that the patient told us. Then we have allergies, genetics and other lofty explanations—valid in many cases—which can compete with some heavenly influence (influenza), or bad air (malaria), or plain and simple *Karmas*.

We label them as *primary, essential, or idiopathic,* indicating that we have not gotten the slightest idea what it is.

1. *Primary* means it is not due to or *secondary* to anything that we can think of.
2. *Essential* takes us to the abstract fundamental things that exist thanks to nothing else but themselves, that is, they are the *cause* and they are the *effects*.
3. With *idiopathic*, we go to the extreme and blame our patients for having something that even we cannot diagnose. Literally, it means *one's own (idio-) trouble (pathy)*.

We are not the only ones to pull wool over people's eyes and over ours as well, at our own peril. I like it when we say, *fever of unknown origin*. At least we are being honest and we intend to do something about that fever.

I often wonder, who is the best, a modern spiritual authority performing miracles, or a magician, or a con man? The last is a crook and cheats everybody outright, without making any claims. There are many so-called saints, who use some ill understood phenomenon to justify his (I think I can leave *her* out) sainthood. He is lying, too.

Magician is the only one who tells us outright that he is tricking us. He insists that no matter how real his miracles may appear to be, they are simply deceptions. (S)he is the only honest one. Mother nature or the Almighty above is the real magician, showing us all kinds of tricks, making us believe in them, reminding us repeatedly that we are wrong in believing our eyes and ears.

That is what makes the research wonderful. In it, we let ourselves to be made fun of, be made fools of ourselves, believing every now and then that finally, we have uncovered all His or Her secrets. We have possessed the virgin Saraswati, who knows well who has possessed whom.

During an ASAIO meeting after I had returned to MPC again, a smart woman who had befriended me, sitting at our dining table, looked at my identification badge and reading it out loud mumbled,

"Manhattan *Psychiatric* Center! Dr. Shah, what *are* you working with, the artificial *brain*, or what?"

"No, the same old one that I was born with!" I replied. We are no way near the artificial brain. Fifty years ago, we could have said the same about all the artificial organs and intelligence that we take it for granted today.

That is the journey from the unknown to the commonplace, from the terra incognita to the territory well known, too well known to us, to remain wonderful. Searching for wonder in that, what research is all about.

There are only two territories. One is terra incognita or the unknown territory. The other is the territory that is already known, or we think we do know. Even though we may be dead wrong in our assumption, its knowledge does work in our day-to-day life. Isn't that wonderful!

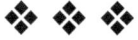

QUESTIONS,

ANSWERS,

AND

EXCLAMATIONS

FROM THE GARAGE OF A CLINICAL RESEARCHER

PART: II

REJECTIONS' HALL OF FAME!

The second part contains unpublished papers as such, current as of the date they were last amended. Their date of writing can be guessed by looking at the latest reference quoted in that paper. Since these are the latest versions, their very first versions may have preceded them by tens of years. The future researchers would have to bring these to the standards prevailing in their times.

Unlike in part: I, in this part I have not listed the take home points. Discussion section of a particular paper does go into that. I have intentionally avoided enumerating the journals that had rejected these papers. They are not presented here for the reader to judge whether journals were justified in rejecting them. I am sure they were. That is not the point now. What is intended is for someone to get the idea, develop it properly or differently and make it work for maybe another purpose. I hope to generate the proverbial light, not heat.

All work presented here was approved by appropriate research committees of various hospitals and medical colleges.

PART: II
REJECTIONS' HALL OF FAME!

★★★

30. WATER INDUCED VARIABILITY OF RELATIONSHIP BETWEEN BODY TEMPERATURE AND HEART RATE IN HEALTHY VOLUNTEERS[27]

Bharat S. Shah, M.D.
Assistant Professor of Medicine

ABSTRACT

Background: Heart rate is a directly linear function of body temperature (Liebermeister's Rule). An investigation of exceptions to this rule suggested that the relationship is affected by the water balance.

Method: Five adult volunteers were studied under ad libitum water intake, forced intake, and under water deprivation. Deep body temperature (BT), heart rate (HR), water intake, urine osmolality, and systemic blood pressure were recorded.

Results: The algebraic value of the product of the change in body temperature and that in the heart rate ($\Delta BT \times \Delta HR$) became more negative with forced water intake, and more positive with water deprivation. It correlated ($p<0.05$, or better) with intake, and urinary osmolality. ΔHR was found to be a direct or an inverse function of ΔBT, depending upon whether the urinary osmolality was high or low respectively.

Conclusions: Relationship between BT and HR is a variable one, modulated by water balance. The Liebermeister relationship occurs under water deficit, a mirror-image type under water excess, and a "Mixed" type, or "Other," under rela-

---

27   From the Department of Medicine, Coler Memorial Hospital affiliation of the New York Medical College, Valhalla, NY.

tively normal water balance. This observation has physiological, pathophysiological, and clinical implications.

Citation: *Shah BS.*
Water induced variability of relationship between body temperature and heart rate in healthy volunteers. In
Questions, Answers, and Exclamations from the Garage of a Clinical Researcher. P. 169 - 188, 2011 Setubandh Publications, New York.

Key Words:

Typhoid fever   Relative Bradycardia
Physical Diagnosis   Thermoregulation
Premenstrual Syndrome   Homeostasis
Legionnaire's Disease

INTRODUCTION

Tachycardia associated with fever (figure: 1, top) was noticed long before the invention of either a practical watch or the thermometer. Herophilus (3rd century B.C.), who first used the word "pulse" as it is understood today, was also aware of it (18). Falconer, in 1796 proposed (3) grading of fevers according to the degree of accompanying tachycardia. Wünderlich (24) wrote, "A Manual of Medical Thermometry," and his contemporary Liebermeister (11) in the 1860s formally stated the now famous rule that the mean pulse rate increases by eight beats per minute per degree Celsius rise in body temperature (Liebermeister relationship-LMR, hereafter). In the 125 plus years that have elapsed, no explanation for this rule has been offered.

There are conditions in which the increase in the pulse rate is less than that expected according to the rule ("relative bradycardia"), e.g., typhoid fever (17), viral hepatitis, Legionnaire's disease

(22), etc. At times, no definite relationship is observed (figure: 1, middle), thereby raising questions about the basic physiological relationship, if any at all, between body temperature and heart rate.

The present author reported (19) a reciprocal or mirror-image relationship (MIR hereafter) in five patients. MIR is characterized by an increase in temperature associated with a decrease in heart rate and vice versa, quite the opposite of the LMR. The cause of MIR and how it relates to the LMR are not known.

Preliminary work done in 50 patients (unpublished data) revealed that temperature and heart rate displayed both, LMR and MIR, shifting from one kind to the other and back (figure: 1, middle panel), their daily frequency correlating well with the ambient temperature and relative humidity, thereby suggesting the possible influence water balance. Similarity of findings in all patients indicated that both phenomena are possibly physiological. Consequently, behavior of heart rate with respect to physiological temperatures was studied in healthy volunteers under various amount of water intake.

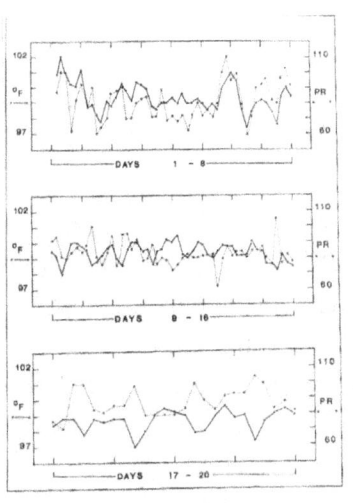

Figure: 1. Continuous plot of body temperature (BT) and pulse rate (PR) covering a patient's twenty-day hospital stay, redrawn from clinical records, for illustration. Note the expanded scale for days 17-20. Data were recorded very four hours (midnight, 4 and 8 am, noon, 4 and 8 pm). Several such observations prompted the present study.

In the top panel, the patient had a few temperature elevations, and BT and PR either both increased or both decreased (LMR, Liebermeister relationship). In the middle panel, BT has come down somewhat and most data points still show LMR. A few begin to show an increase in either BT or PR with a decrease in the other (MIR, mirror-image relationship), together with LMR, i.e., a "Mixed" type relationship, or the "Other." In the bottom panel, BT decreases with an increase in PR in morning, to be reversed later in the day. This panel shows predominantly MIR. Circadian rhythmicity strongly suggested in this panel could not be confirmed. PR on days 16-20 inversely correlated with BT (not shown).

MATERIALS AND METHODS

Five nonsmoker adult volunteers (table: 1), two men and three women, able to do their everyday activities, were studied. Each subject was studied under different water intake on three nonconsecutive days throughout the year, in a centrally air conditioned room. On other days, the subjects led their normal lives. Dry and wet bulb room temperatures were recorded initially, midway through, and at the end of the studies.

Serial #	Sex	Age	Weight in lbs	Intake In mls	% of Pro-posed
1	F	28	85	1290	63.98
2	M	33	149	3060	113.83
3	F	39	173	2580	95.98
4	M	23	223	2640	98.2
5	F	30	105.5	1980	98.82

Table: 1. Personal data on volunteers. F: Female, M: Male. Forced water intake between 11 am and 2 p.m. Is shown. For details on "proposed," see "Methods."

The study subjects did not eat or drink after the midnight before the studies. They reported at 8.00 am, changed into light clothing, then reclined in a bed with its head elevated by 45° to avoid discomfort, and for constant cardiac position for electrocardiographic recording. They were awake throughout, with eyes open, and they engaged in neutral conversation with the author, whom they knew well.

They were given cool tap water without ice, salt, or sweetener. Water was allowed to stand for five minutes to remove excess air. Temperature of ingested food, even before it is swallowed, elicits (7) hypothalamic thermoregulatory responses. No food, drugs, or beverages were given. Water intake was recorded. When the subjects had an option of whether to drink, they were actually given a glass of water in their hands, then they decided whether and how much to drink. This was to avoid voluntary dehydration (2).

(a) *Forced Intake:* Before readings of body temperature, heart rate, and blood pressure were taken at 9.00 am, after the subjects were weighed having emptied their urinary bladder. They stayed without any water until 11.00 am. From 11.00 am through 2.00 pm, they were given water every 15 minutes, depending upon their body weights, viz., 6 oz. (180 ml) if they weighed 125 lbs. or less, and 8 oz. (240 ml), if more. They were given 12 such potions, and were encouraged to take more water. A very large intake in one dose generates sudomotor responses (4). After 2.00 pm, the subjects excreted the water until conclusion at 4.00 pm.

(b) *Ad Libitum Intake:* After the baseline readings were taken at 9.00 am, the subjects stayed without any water until 11.00 am. From 11.00 am through 4.00 pm, the subjects took water as they desired.

(c) *Water Deprivation:* Baseline readings were taken at 9.00 am. No water was given until 2.00 pm. Then it was given ad libitum until conclusion at 4.00 pm.

Thus in three studies, water loading and excretion of water load, ad libitum intake, water deprivation and replenishment were included.

Deep body (core) temperature was recorded every half an hour with a deep body thermometer (Ambulatory Monitoring, Ardsley, NY) via a chest plate affixed with an adhesive tape to the sternal area to avoid the discomfort (and change in heart rate) associated with rectal probes. The plate generates heat which then equilibrates with the body core. The instrument displays the core temperature computed from the heat transfer between the plate and the body core. The readings are in tenths of a degree Celsius. They were recorded manually.

The heart rate was recorded half hourly from the integrated signal of a cardiac monitor with a digital display. On a visual signal from a timer, the heart rate was read first, then the temperature was recorded. Automated recording gave spurious data because of even minor movements by the subjects for positioning, etc. Therefore, manual recording was resorted to. Neither the signal from the timer, nor the displays of temperature and heart rate were visible to the subjects, thereby to avoid the biofeedback. If the display was changing, then a mean of the readings was recorded.

Systemic blood pressure was recorded every half an hour with an Arteriosonde (® Ross Medical Instruments) recorder, triggered manually after the above data were gathered. Then the subjects were asked to get out of bed to empty the urinary bladder as completely as possible, at the bedside. Urine volume was recorded and a sample was refrigerated for determination of osmolality by freezing point method. A standard 12 lead electrocardiogram was taken every hour, after all the above readings were taken. All these procedures were over within 12-15 minutes.

DEFINITIONS AND ANALYSES

Changes in body temperature (ΔBT) and that in heart rate (ΔHR) were calculated for each 30-minute interval and their relationship was classified as under:

(i)   LMR, when BT and HR, either both increased or both decreased,

(ii)   MIR, when one increased and the other decreased, and

(iii) "Other," or "Mixed," when BT, or HR, or both remain unchanged, i.e., $\Delta BT < 0.1°C$ or $\Delta HR < 1/\text{min}$.

The product $\Delta BT \times \Delta HR$ was computed for each reading.
A positive value of the product indicates LMR, a negative one
MIR, and zero indicates "other." The product was plotted as a dependent variable against water intake, urine output, their difference, cumulated difference, urinary osmolality, and blood pressure
as independent variables. ΔHR was plotted as a function of ΔBT,
keeping the urinary osmolality constant at more than and less than
280 mOsmol/L.

Although the data were gathered every 30 minutes (except
the electrocardiograms), hourly data points were analyzed to avoid
observer bias. Linear Regression analyses were done using the
Least Square method. Regression coefficient "r" was calculated
and two-tail probabilities were computed ('p' values). "Student" t-
test was used for significance of difference between two mean values for paired data.

OBSERVATIONS AND RESULTS
Subject # 5 could not come for the water deprivation study
because of her involvement in an automobile accident with resultant chronic problems requiring medications. So, 14 studies were
done in five volunteers. Forced intake did not induce headache,
chest pain, diaphoresis, or dyspnoea. Subject # 1 could take only
64% of the proposed intake, and vomited once. No more water was
given, but the observations were continued and results are presented herein. All others took water as proposed, or more (table: 1).
They felt hungry on the days of ad libitum intake and of deprivation.

The electrocardiograms did not show any changes in the ST
segments, or electrical axes. No arrhythmias were observed. The
amplitude of various cardiographic waves showed striking changes

with varying water intake, and these are being reported separately[28].

The ambient temperature (dry bulb) varied between 70.2 - 75.3 °F, the wet bulb reading was 54.5 - 63.2 °F, and the barometer read 29.58 to 30.47" of Hg, during the whole period. The daily variations were 3 °F, 1.6 °F, and 0.2" at the most, respectively. Water temperature was 60 - 65 °F on various days, but was nearly unchanged on any particular day.

Table: 2 shows the data on different variables. With forced intake, diastolic BP increased, urinary osmolality fell and body weight increased. With deprivation, the weight decreased, and the osmolality increased further. All subjects lost some weight with water deprivation and ad libitum intake, attributable to starvation, partly compensated for by some water retention.

Interelationship of BT and HR:

BT and HR both showed diurnal variations (compare "end" with "control" on all three days, table: 2). The peak procedure BT increased with ad libitum intake and with deprivation, but fell with forced intake. The HR, on the contrary, continuously increased on all days, i.e., BT dissociated from HR with forced intake. LMR and MIR both occurred on all three days, the former tended to be more common with water deprivation and high urine osmolality, while the latter with the forced intake and ad libitum intake, both with a low osmolality (peak procedure, table: 2).

Effect of Water on $\Delta BT \times \Delta HR$:

The product of change in BT and that in HR in one hour, $\Delta BT \times \Delta HR$, separates LMR from MIR by its positive and negative values respectively. As shown in figure: 2, the forced water intake makes the mean value of the product more negative, depri-

---

[28] See the next paper.

vation makes it more positive, while the ad libitum intake makes it sequentially both, negative and positive.

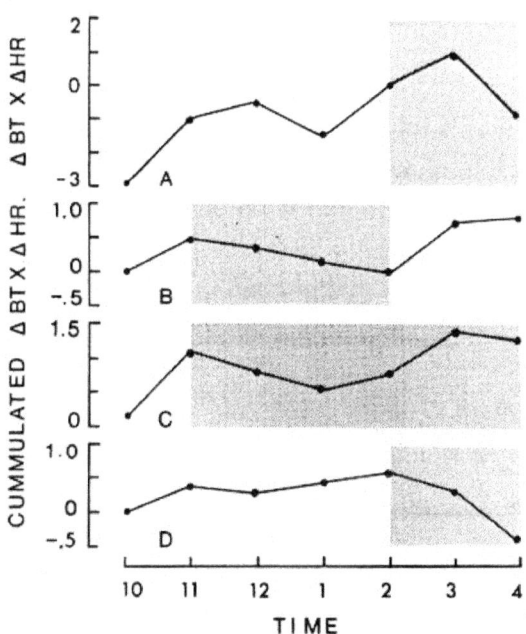

Figure: 2. Plots B, C, and D show the effect of water intake and deprivation on the mean (of all subjects) cumulated ΔBT X ΔHR, taking the control value as zero. With water deprivation (unshaded areas) the cumulated product became more positive. With water intake (plot: B, 11-2 p.m., with forced intake; plot: D, 2-4 p.m. after deprivation) it became more negative, while it became more negative and then more positive sequentially with ad libitum water intake (plot: C, 11 am - 4 p.m.).
Plot: A shows the effect of water deprivation on the product ΔBT X ΔHR (hourly, actual value, not cumulated) in a woman (subject # 1) who was one day premenstrual. All points from 10 am - 2 p.m. show a negative value of the product (also, see figure: 5) despite water deprivation, i.e., MIR, instead of LMR. However, the trend is towards less and less negative value, showing that hydration is more important than intake per se.

Table: 2.   DATA ON ALL SUBJECTS UNDER
DIFFERENT STATES OF HYDRATION.

Variables.		Forced Intake.		Ad Libitum Intake.		Water Deprivation.	
Intake		2310	(688.04)	510.6	(155.71)	000	(000)
Output		1114	(615.82)	636.6	(155.06)	179	(82.04)
Osmolality	C.	448.2	(356.7) AC	534.2	(217.05) ABC	591.0	(285.45)
	P.	55.4	(9.86)	125.4	(52.12)	707.0	(213.14)
	E.	172.2	(121.84)	224	(130.69)	163.25	(65.39)
BP Syst	C.	112.4	(9.91)	105.4	(14.41)	113	(8.71)
	P.	111.2	(7.29)	103.6	(12.93)	105.25	(12.68)
	E.	107.8	(2.77)	108.6	(9.86)	109.0	(12.96)
BP Diast	C.	72.8	(6.57) A	67.8	(6.61)	75.5	(9.98)
	P.	80.4	(5.07)	70.4	(14.08)	69	(16.71)
	E.	76.4	(7.73)	72.4	(9.91)	71	(10.98)
BT oC	C.	36.98	(0.4)	36.68	(0.48)	36.33	(0.64)
	P.	36.75	(0.52)	36.94	(0.46)	36.71	(0.54)
	E.	37.1	(0.20)	36.98	(0.36)	36.77	(0.38)
HR/Min.	C.	64.2	(6.34)	64	(8.39)	59	(14.87)
	P.	66.4	(8.08)	66	(12.70)	59.52	(13.88)
	E.	68.8	(7.66)	66.8	(13.44)	63.75	(18.94)
Frequen.	LMR	3		4		5	
	MIR	7		7		3	
	OTHER	5		4		4	
Weight	C.	146.4	(54.4)	150.2	(52.2)	161.37	(51.37)
	P.	148.6	(55.62)	149.7	(52.10)	159.0	(52.84)
	E.	146.3	(54.6)	149.4	(52.43)	159.0	(54.12)

Table: 2 Data on different variables (mean ± SD) with various water intakes. In case of water deprivation, only four subjects were studied (see "Results"). Intake and urine output data refer to 11 am to 2 p.m.. "Control" reading (C) for BT, HR, BP, and Osmolality is at 10 am, "end" (E) is at 4 p.m., and "Peak" is at 2 p.m. Letters after the numbers indicate A: Difference between the mean control and the mean peak values significant at 5% level, or better. B: The same between the control and the end values, and C: The same between the peak and the end values. "Frequen" is Frequency, HR/min is Heart rate per minute, BP syst and Diast mean Blood Pressure, Systolic and Diastolic.

Table: 3.   EFFECT OF SEVERAL WATER VARIABLES ON ΔBT X ΔHR.

Water	Sub	N =	Intake	Output	I - O	Cum (I-O)	Osm	Syst.	Diast.	Mean	Pulse Pressure
Forced	1	6	-.37	-.58							
	2	7	-.79 (5)		-.67	-.51					
	3	7	-.38	-.53			.80				
	4	7	-.46	-.65		-.84 (2)	.76				
	5	7	-.52	-.35	-.47	-.43					
Ad Lib	1	5					.41	-.92 (5)	.42	-.80 (10)	-.95 (2)
	2	7						.91(1)	.67		-.72 (10)
Deprvd	2	6		-.96(1)		.76 (10)	.67				.46
	3	7	-.63								
	4	7		-.42	-.44	.48			.45	.36	-.30

Table: 3. Regression of hourly ΔBT X ΔHR on different independent variables under various water intakes. Two digit numbers are "r" values, minus sign (-) indicates an inverse correlation, the rest indicate a directly linear correlation. Blanks and subjects not shown indicate no correlation, i.e., r = < ± 0.30. The numbers in the parentheses are "p" values.

In each subject, on one or more days, ΔBT X ΔHR showed (table: 3) statistically significant correlations with the corresponding water variables and the blood pressure. It was an inversely linear function of intake (also, see figure: 3) and of systolic BP, and a directly linear one of urinary osmolality (also, figure: 4) and of diastolic BP. other correlations were more variable.

***

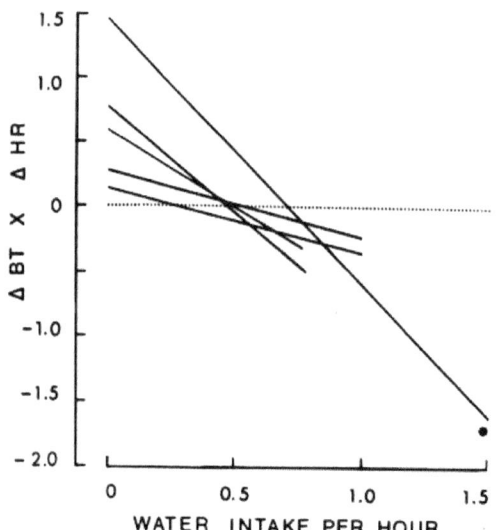

Figure: 3. $\Delta BT \times \Delta HR$ is inversely related to the corresponding water intake. Regression lines are shown for all subjects, under forced water intake. High intake is associated with a lower or negative value of the product (i.e., MIR). The asterisk (*) indicates $p<0.05$. The area above the horizontal axis is LMR, below it is MIR, while the data points falling on the horizontal axis would represent the "other," wherein BT and/ or HR remained unchanged.

Figure: 4. $\Delta BT \times \Delta HR$ shows a directly linear relationship with urinary osmolality. LMR, MIR, and "other" same as in figure: 3. Regression lines for all subjects are shown. Positive value of the product (LMR) occurs in association with high urinary osmolality,   while negative value (MIR) occurs with low osmolality. The asterisk (*) indicates $p<0.05$.

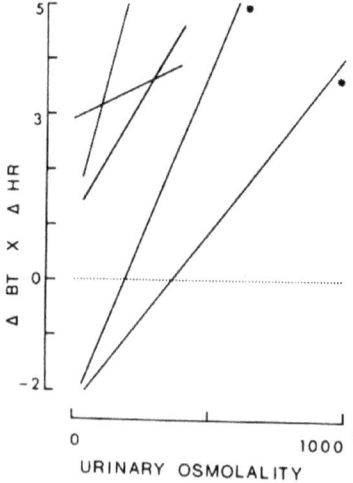

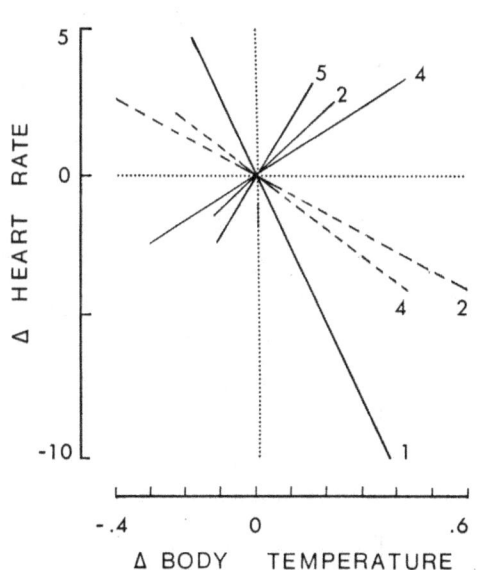

Figure: 5. Regression of ΔHR over ΔBT is a "seesaw," being directly or inversely linear depending upon whether the urinary osmolality is more (solid lines) or less (broken lines) than 280 mOsmol/L, respectively. Upper right and lower left quadrants represent LMR, the other two quadrants represent MIR. The axes represent "other."

The numbers refer to the subjects. Pooled data from three days in each subject. Note that in subject # 2 and # 4, the correlation of ΔHR over ΔBT changes from direct to inverse on lowering the urinary osmolality. Correlations with r ≤ ±0.30 are not shown. To facilitate the comparison of slopes, all regression lines are drawn through the origin.

ΔHR as a function of ΔBT:

As such, hourly ΔHR correlated poorly with ΔBT (not shown), but when data were subdivided in each subject, according to whether the concurrent urinary osmolality was more, or less than 280 mOsmol/L (approximately same as the normal serum osmolality), a significant relationship emerged (figure; 5). With osmolality > 280 mOsmol/L, ΔHR was found to be a directly linear function of ΔBT, indicating LMR, in three of the four subjects. In the fourth one (#1), it was inversely linear, indicating MIR. That subject was one-day premenstrual (last menstrual period: 28 days, she started having her period the same evening) on the day of water deprivation, the day that contributed seven of the eight data points (figure; 2). With osmolality < 280 mOsmol/L, in all subjects, ΔBT X ΔHR was found to be an inverse function of ΔBT X ΔHR, i.e., MIR.

DISCUSSION

Heart rate increases linearly with an increase in the body temperature (LMR) caused by fevers (24, 11), hot water baths (10), exposure to warm environment (8), or exercise (23). One factor common to all these is the water deficit that all these can cause. The water loss accompanying the evaporative heat loss, especially in febrile patients studied by Liebermeister (11) could be enormous. In the present study also, the LMR occurred with low water intake (figure: 3), high urinary osmolality (figure: 4, 5), and other conditions associated with a relative lack of water (table: 3). The data strongly suggest that LMR is associated with water deficit.

When the subjects were water loaded, as indicated by high intake (table: 3), resultant high urinary output, more water retention (In-Out), low urinary osmolality, high systolic and low diastolic blood pressure, the BT and HR displayed MIR, instead of the conventional LMR. Thus, LMR is not only associated with a relative lack of water, but it even depends upon it; the relationship between BT and HR is a "seesaw" influenced by water—LMR with water deficit, and MIR with water excess (figure: 5).

Exercising in presence of experimental dehydration is known to increase the heart rate further for a given body temperature (14), indicating that the slope of the regression line of HR over BT is increased by dehydration, and is decreased by water replenishment (4) or by overhydration (14). No mirror-image relationship was observed in the latter study, probably because the MIR depends upon an absolute water excess, while overhydration in exercising subjects may amount to nothing more than "less dehydration."

It is the state of hydration rather than the amount of water intake per se that is important. The volunteer who was premenstrual, showed (figure: 2, 5) an inverse correlation between ΔHR and ΔBT despite the urinary osmolality being more than 280 mOsmol/L, and despite the water deprivation, instead of showing a direct correlation as did the rest of the subjects. This might be due to the premenstrual retention of water (16, 21), high urinary osmolality being a "cause," or mechanism of water retention, rather than a result of water deficit.

In the present study, BT and HR were recorded periodically, thereby making them time series data, hence, derivatives of BT and HR were analyzed instead of plotting HR against BT, unlike in the other studies cited. With severe and sustained overhydration in clinical situations (e.g., data from figure: 1, bottom panel), HR did correlate inversely (not shown) with BT. Significant overhydration cannot be produced and maintained in the healthy volunteers without administering hormones, etc.

Occurrence of LMR and MIR cannot be ascribed to chance alone (19). HR is affected by many extraneous factors which were controlled as far as possible (see "Methods"). Heart rate variability, as it is affected by respiratory rate, blood pressure, and body temperature, has been reviewed recently by Pieper et al (15). Diurnal and circadian rhythms of HR and BT (12, 9) increase both these in the afternoon, and therefore, cannot explain the occurrence of MIR, in which one variable increases while the other decreases. One possible mechanism is that water, by its thermal capacity may lower the core temperature, stimulating thermogenesis and metabolism, and may increase the heart rate by Bainbridge reflex (1) and other mechanisms. During the excretion of water load the conditions are restored.

Harrison et al (6) discussed the relative effects of body fluid volume and tonicity on BT and HR, but not on the interrelationship of the latter two. There are several receptors (20), hypothalamic centers (13), antiduretic and other hormones, natriuretic factors (5), etc., which may participate in mediating the effect of water, but our data do not permit further comments on these.

Whatever the purpose and mechanism of production of LMR and MIR, both these kinds of relationships occur in a wide range of physiological and pathophysiological (19) conditions. "Normal" state of hydration varies from minor water deficit to minor water excess, hence, it may be associated with a mixture of LMR and MIR (figure: 1, middle). The relationship called "Other" (when BT and/or HR remain unchanged, see "Methods"), mathematically falling between LMR and MIR (figure: 3, 4) also probably represents euhydration.

Since LMR and MIR each can occur under the state of euhydration, it is the preponderance in frequency and magnitude (figure: 3, 4, and figure: 1, top and bottom) that are important. The higher values of the product correlates with the more extreme conditions of hydration.

In view of the flattening effect of excess water on the "see-saw" of the regression line of HR on BT, one could hypothesize that the "relative bradycardia" observed in typhoid fever (17), Legionnaire"s disease (22), and brain tumors (17) is caused by intracranial, or systemic, or both water logging.

In viral hepatitis, the water logging may trigger the similar or intraabdominal water-sensitive receptors (6). Typhoid fever and Legionnaire's disease both also manifest by an abdominal illness. These conditions are probably associated with a relative water excess which causes the concurrent relative bradycardia. Data are needed to explore this hypothesis.

Data are presented to show that in healthy volunteers, interrelationship of body temperature and heart rate is variable, modulated by the state of hydration. The Liebermeister relationship is contingent upon water deficit, and is replaced by a mirror-image one in presence of water excess. A mixture of these two represents euhydration.

In clinical situations, various kinds of relationships can serve as noninvasive indicators of state of hydration, to be verified by conventional methods. It is hypothesized that relative bradycardia of typhoid fever, Legionnaire's disease, etc., is caused by a relative water excess. Liebermeister's rule has bee revisited, explained, and expanded.

Acknowledgements: The author expresses his gratitude to Dr. Sunil Amerasinghe for technical help.

BIBLIOGRAPHY

1.   Bainbridge FA.
     The Influence of venous filling upon rate of heart.
     J. Physiol. 50: p. 65, 1915.
2.   Bar-or O, Dotan R, Inbar O, Zonder H.
     Voluntary dehydration in 10- to 12-year-old boys.
     J. Appl. Physiol; Respire. Environ. Exercise Physiol. 1980. 48(1); 104-108.
3.   Falconer W., in Observations respecting the pulse intended to point out with clear certainty, the indications which it signifies especially in feverish complaints, p. 50, Cadell, Jr., London.
4.   Goetz KL.
     Atrial receptors, natriuretic peptides, and the kidney—current understanding.
     Mayo Clin. Proc. 61:600-603, 1986.
5.   Greenleaf JE, Castle BL.
     Exercise temperature regulation in man during hypohydration and hyperhydration.
     J. Appl. Physiol. 1971, 30(6): 847-853.
6.   Harrison MH, Edwards RJ, Fennesy PA.
     Intravenous volume and tonicity as factors in regulation of body temperature,
     J. Appl. Physiol: Respirat. Environ. Exercise Physiol. 44: 69-75, 1978.

7.   Hayward JN, Baker MA.
Role of cerebral arterial blood in the regulation of brain temperature in the monkey.
Am. J. Of Physiology 1968, 215(2): 389-403.

8.   Horseman DH, Horvath SM.
Cardiovascular and temperature regulatory changes during progressive dehydration and euhydration.
J. Appl. Physiol. 33(4): 446-450, 1972.

9.   Kawasaki T, Mistook M, Halberg E, Halberg F.
Circadian and circatriginatan rhythms in pulse, oral temperature and blood pressure of clinically healthy Japanese women.
Chronobiologia, 5: 399-406, 1978.

10.   Lemonnier S. As quoted by
Liebermeister C., in
Handbuch der pathologie und therapie des fiebers. P. 461, F. Vogal (Leipzig), 1875.

11.   Liebermeister C., in
Handbuch der pathologie und therapie des fiebers. P. 460-467, F. Vogal (Leipzig), 1875.

12.   Marietta H, Timbal J.
Clinical circadian rhythm of temperature in man. Comparative study with two experimental protocols.
Chronobiologia, 8:87-100, 1981.

13.   Morishima MS, Gale CC.
Relationship of blood pressure and heart rate to body temperature in baboons.
Am. J. Physiol. 223(2): 387-395. 1972.

14.   Nadel ER, Fortney SM, Wenger CB.
Effect of hydration state on circulatory and thermal regulations.
J. Appl. Physiol: Respirat. Environ. Exercise Physiol. 49(4): 715-721, 1980.

15. Pieper S, Hammil S.
    Heart rate variability: Technique and investigational applications in cardiovascular medicine.
    Mayo Clin Proc 1995; 70: 995-964.

16. Reid RL, Yen SS.
    Premenstrual syndrome.
    Am. J. Of Obst. Gynecology. 139: 85-104, 1981.

17. Sahli H, in
    A treatise on diagnostic methods of examination. Edited by N. B. Potter, second edition, translated from the fifth German edition, p. 111.
    W. B. Saunders Company, Philadelphia, 1916.

18. Schone H.
    Markellinus Pulselehre. Fester. 49. Versamml. Dutch.
    Philogen U. Schulman 1907, p. 448, as quoted by
    Boas EP, Goldsmidt EF. In
    The Pulse Rate, p. 4, Charles C. Thomas, Springfield, IL, USA 1932.

19. Shah BS.
    Mirror-image relationship between body temperature and pulse rate.
    JAMA 1979, 242: p. 2760.

20. Skoreki KL, Brannier BM.
    Body fluid homeostasis in man. A comparative review.
    Am. J. Med. 70: 77-88, 1981.

21. Steiner M., Carrol BJ.
    The psychobiology of premenstrual dysphoria. Review of theories and treatment.
    Psychoneuroendocrinology, 2: 321-335, 1977.

22. Tsai TF, Finn DR, Pilkaytis BD, McCauley W, Martin SM, and Fraser DW
    Legionnaire's disease: Clinical features of epidemic in Philadelphia.

23.   Wesley K, There R.

Der Kreislauf Imo Dinettes der Warmeregulation.

Z. Ges. Expl. Med. 112: 345-379, 1943, as quoted by,

There R., in Handbook of Physiology, Circulation, Section: 2, Vol. III, p. 1946.

Hamilton F, Editor. American Physiological Society, Washington D. C., 1965.

24.   Wunderlich CA, in

On the temperature in diseases. A manual of medical thermometry.

Translated from the second German edition by

Woodman WB, p. 213, The New Sydenham Society, London, 1871.

31. EFFECT OF VARYING ORAL WATER INTAKE ON THE AMPLITUDE OF ELECTROCARDIOGRAM OF HEALTHY VOLUNTEERS[29]

Bharat S. Shah, M.D.
Asst. Professor of Medicine

ABSTRACT

Background: EKG amplitude is affected by many variables, viz., heart rate, effusions around the heart, etc., but the state of hydration per se is not known to be one of these. An incidental observation of changes in the EKG amplitude occurring during a study of forced water intake led to this experimental study.

Methods: Five adult volunteers were studied under ad libitum water intake, forced intake, and water deprivation. Twelve lead EKG were recorded every hour, and mean amplitude of the three tallest QRS complexes in each lead was computed. That was plotted against the hourly cumulated intake minus output, and regression analysis was done.

Results: Amplitude of almost all EKG waves correlated significantly ($p<0.05$, or better) with the Cum(In-Out). When the changes were grossly appreciable (without measurements), P and T waves were flattened with water excess, while the Q, R, and S waves were either augmented or flattened. The PR interval, ST segment, electrical axes, or the electrical position of the heart did not change.

Conclusions: Water-induced changes in the EKG amplitude, observed in five healthy volunteers, were attributed to the changes in the end-diastolic volume, and in electrical conductivity of the intracardiac blood (Brody's effect), with a

---

29 From the Dept. of Medicine and Gerontology. Coler Memorial Hospital affiliation of New York Medical College, Valhalla, NY.

resultant increase in the inhomogeneity of the thoracic volume conductor.

Citation: *Shah BS.*

Effect of varying oral water intake on the amplitude of electrocardiogram of healthy volunteers. In Questions, Answers, and Exclamations from the Garage of a Clinical Researcher. P. 189 - 205, 2011 Setubandh Publications, New York.

Key Words:
Brody's Effect
Urinary Osmolality
Thorax - Inhomogeneity of

Hemodilution
End-diastolic Volume

INTRODUCTION

Amplitude of various electrocardiographic (EKG) waves is known to be affected by several factors (8). It also varies from day to day, and even on the same day. It is not known to be affected by the state of hydration of the body.

Following Comroe's advice (6), I would tell the reason for this study "as it was." During a pilot experiment for a study of effect of water on body temperature—heart rate relationship[30], with myself as a guinea pig, a lay friend and assistant of mine was impressed by the reduction in the "size" (amplitude) of the tracing on the cardiac monitor. Being painfully aware of the capacity of cardiac monitors to do various things, including showing a straight line, I would have ordinarily ignored this observation. I had reasons not to.

The temperature-heart rate study had come about thanks to my inability to dismiss a mirror-image relationship as a chance

---

[30] See the previous paper.

event (19), thereby reaffirming the respect for such "chance" events. That, combined with my interest in artificial lungs (22), had led me to a paper by Spence (21) in the Transactions of the ASAIO, in which the author had used the water-induced changes in the bioelectrical impedance to an introduced electric current as an indicator of body water in hemodialysis patients.

The rest followed by itself. Instead of introducing the current, we were picking up body's own current as EKG tracing. It made sense. Insulating effect of body water was apparently affecting the amplitude of the EKG, as the pleural and pericardial effusions are known to do. It turned out to be far more complicated and fascinating. This paper reports on the observations and their implications.

MATERIALS AND METHODS

This study was done as a part of another study in which five adult volunteers, able to do their usual activities were studied after an overnight fast, under (1) forced water intake (one glass of water every fifteen minutes, or more water if they could drink it) for two hours, followed by its excretion, (ii) water deprivation, followed by replenishment, and (iii) ad libitum intake, on three different days.

On the day of the study, the subjects wore light clothing and reclined in bed with its head elevated by 45°. Limb leads were attached when needed, to the EKG electrodes which were left in position throughout the study period that day. Positions of precordial leads were marked in ink each day, and a suction cup electrode was used.

A twelve lead standard EKG was taken every hour, for a total of eight EKGs in a day. Each lead was recorded for six or more QRS complexes to include at least one respiratory cycle. Amplitude of QRS complexes was measured with a caliper in standardized manner, and an arithmetic mean of the three tallest complexes in each lead (in each EKG) was computed to avoid the effect of respiratory variation.

Mean EKG amplitude in each lead was plotted as a dependent variable against hourly cumulated water intake minus output, i.e., cumulated (I - O) as the independent variable. Regression analysis by the Least Square method was done. The regression and correlation coefficients and two-tailed probabilities for statistical significance were computed.

OBSERVATIONS AND RESULTS

Subjects were able to take 1290 to 3060 ml of water within three hours on the day of forced intake. They did not complain of chest or stomach discomfort or diaphoresis. Subject # 5 was studied only for two days, as she could not come for the third day because of an automobile accident and subsequent chronic discomfort.

EKGs did not change in their rhythm, electrical axes, transitional zone, PR interval, or QRS duration. ST segments remained isoelectric. Electrical position of the heart did not change. The qualitative changes in the amplitude described below, induced with forced water intake, did not occur in all subjects, and they tended to revert with excretion of excess water. On the day of ad libitum intake and of water deprivation, the changes were less striking; however, quantitatively, the amplitude did correlate significantly with water balance (vide infra).

Qualitative Changes in Various Waves with Forced Intake:

P wave: In most of the subjects, P wave did not show any change. One man (Subject # 2) showed a flattening and disappearance of P wave in lead III with forced intake (figure: 1).

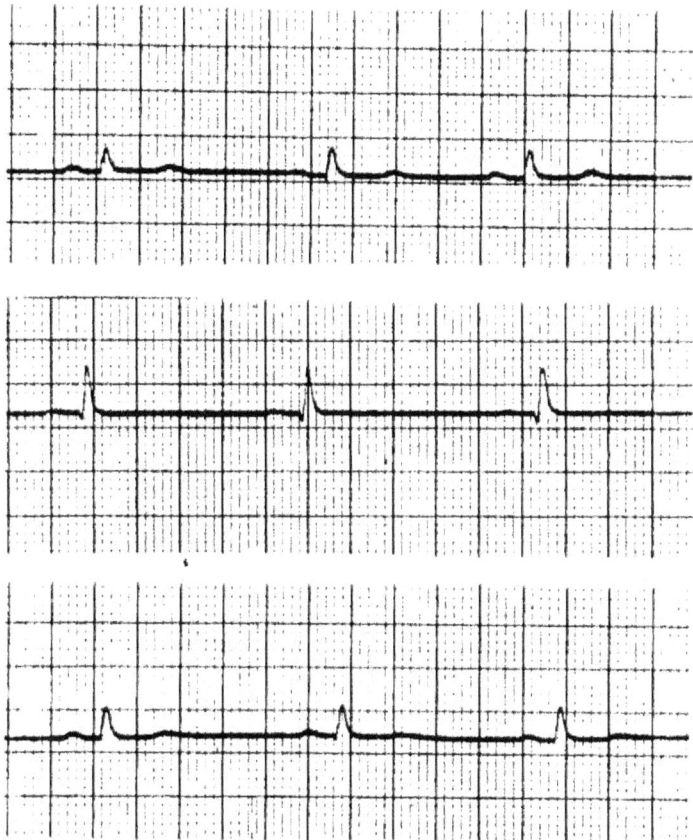

Figure: 1 shows the effect of forced water intake on amplitude of the lead III in a 23 year old man. Figures 1-4 show the control (10 am), peak (2 pm), and end (4 pm) data. EKG strips of the leads indicated were taken at 1 mm = 10 mV standardization. In this figure, the P and T waves nearly disappeared with forced intake, to reappear with excretion of water load. The R wave, on the other hand, got bigger, and then reverted to its original amplitude. The septal q wave deepened temporarily.

Q wave: The septal q wave became more prominent (figure: 1), while the Q wave in aVR in subject # 1 got attenuated (see figure: 2). Other subjects did not show Q wave changes.

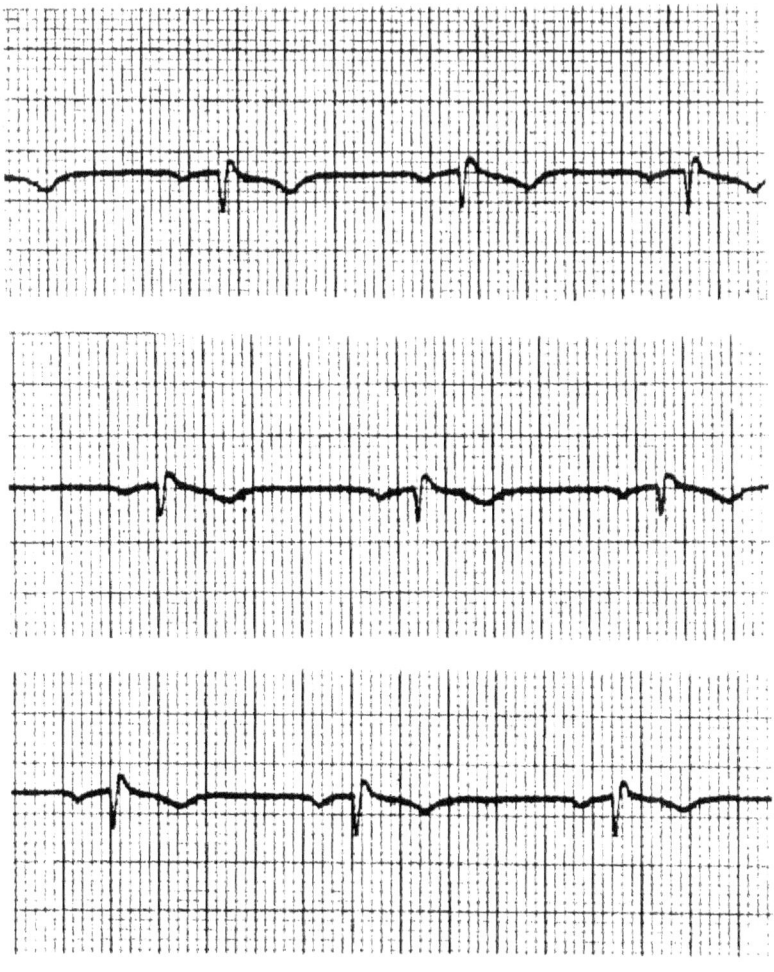

Figure: 2. Lead aVR in a 33 year old man. The Q wave got attenuated with forced intake, then reverted to the control value.

R wave: The R wave (rS or qR) amplitude either increased (figure: 1), or decreased (figure: 3).

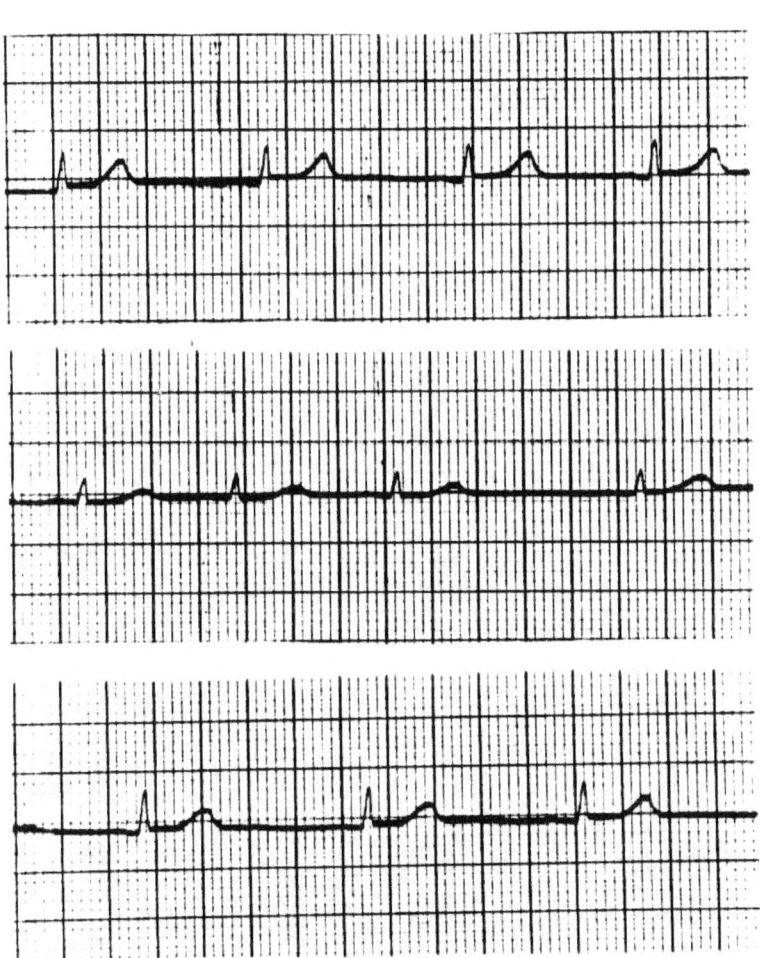

Figure: 3. Lead V₄ in a 30 year old woman. The R and T waves got smaller, while the terminal s wave just appeared in the middle strip temporarily.

S wave: The amplitude of S wave also either increased (figure: 4), or decreased. The terminal s wave (qRs) became prominent (figure: 3).

T wave: The T wave, when it did change, showed flattening (figures: 1, 3). The T wave changes were independent of those
in the QRS complex (figure: 1). In one subject, the T wave changes
were not progressive, but the wave was tallest at the conclusion of
the study at 4 p.m. (figure: 4).

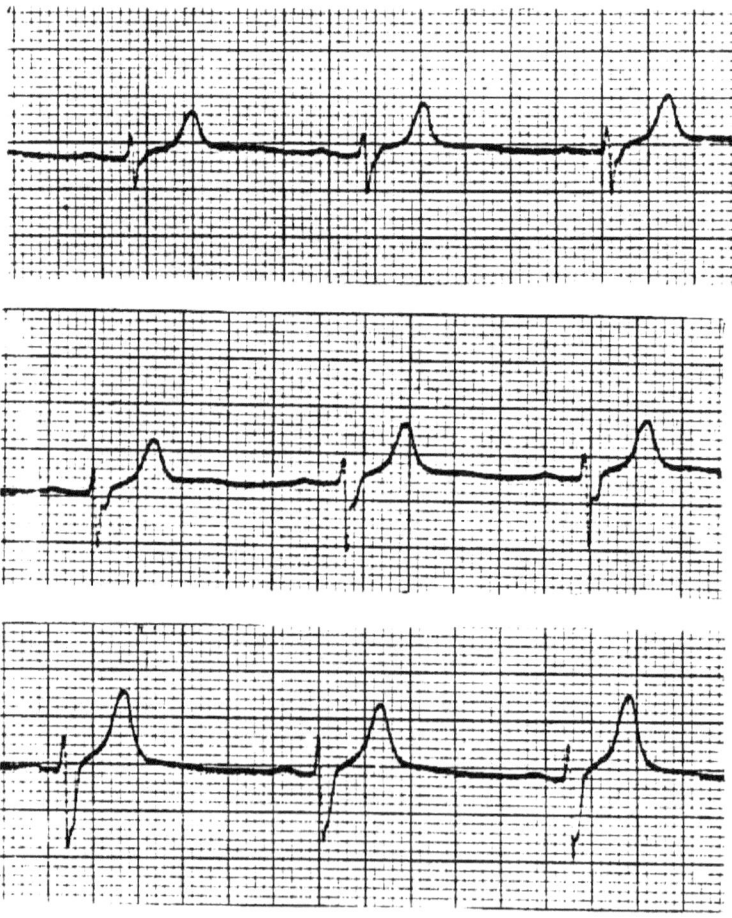

*Figure: 4. Lead V2 in the same volunteer as in figure: 2. The R, and espe-
cially the S waves got augmented and remained so through the end of the
study, when the T wave, unchanged with the forced intake, was then augmented.*

Quantitative QRS Changes:

Unlike the above qualitative changes, those in the QRS amplitude, associated with varying water intake, occurred in all subjects, in most of the leads, on all three days. Table: 1 shows the association of changes in QRS amplitude with the corresponding cumulated (I-O).

TABLE: 1. RELATIONSHIP OF QRS AMPLITUDE WITH CUMMULATIVE WATER INTAKE MINUS OUTPUT.

Subject #	1	2	3	4	5
Sex	M	M	F	F	F
N =	21	21	20	20	14
Lead : 1		+ (1)		— (1)	+
2	—	+ (1)	— (2)	—	— (5)
3	—	+ (1)	— (1)	— (5)	— (2)
aVR	—	+ (1)	—		
aVL		+ (1)	— (1)	— (2)	+ (2)
aVF	—	+ (1)	— (1)		— (1)
V — 1				+	
2	+ (1)			— (5)	—
3		— (1)		— (2)	
4	+	— (1)	—	—	
5		— (1)	—	— (5)	— (1)
6			—		— (1)

Table: 1 shows the results of regression analysis in all subjects, and all EKG leads, for pooled data from three studies under varying water intake in each volunteer. Subject #5 was studied on only two days. Amplitude in each lead (in mm, 1 mV = 10 mm) was the dependent variable, and cumulated (I-O) every hour was the independent variable. (+) indicates a direct, and (—) an inversely linear relationship. The numbers in the parentheses show the level of statistical significance (5 means p<0.05, and so on). Blank spaces indicate no correlation, i.e., r = ± 0.30 or less. N shows the number of data points. Data were pooled because the analysis for individual days done separately showed similar correlations.

TABLE : 2. PRODUCTION OF EKG WAVES BY VARIOUS DIPOLES;
PREDICTED, AND OBSERVED EFFECTS OF INCREASING
THE VOLUME AND/OR CONDUCTIVITY OF INTRACARDIAC
BLOOD.

WAVE	PATTERN	ORIGIN	GENERATING DIPOLES		AMPLITUDE CHANGES	
			RADIAL	TANGENTIAL	PREDICTED	OBSERVED
P		Atrial		*	—	—
Q	qR	Septal	*		+	±
	QS	Sept + RV	*	*	±	±
R	qR	LV	*	*	±	±
	rS	Sept+ RV	*	*	±	±
	rSr'	Terminal LV		*	—	—
S	rS	LV	*	*	±	±
	qRs	Terminal LV		*	—	+
T			?	?	?	—
U			?	?	?	?

Table: 2 compares the changes observed in amplitude of various EKG waves with those predicted according to Brody's effect and the works of scher and Durrer (see Discussion). Radial dipoles are expected to be augmented, while the tangential ones to be attenuated with increased body water and increased conductivity of blood. A "?" denotes unknown information. "Sept" means Septal, RV means Right Ventricular, LV means Left Ventricular. The underlined Patterns indicate the part of the QRS being referred to. The asterisk (*) means "Yes." Attenuation is indicated by a (-), and augmentation by a (+).

DISCUSSION

Influence of volume of intracardiac blood on EKG has been suspected for some time. Lamb (12) challenged the idea that respiratory variations in EKG are due to changes in cardiac position resulting from diaphragmatic movements, and ascribed them instead to the differential filling of the right and left ventricles with phases of respiration. He also noted the transient attenuation of QRS amplitude with tachycardia, and with premature nodal contractions and resultant short diastolic filling periods.

EKG changes during systemic hypervolemia have been studied in intact dogs (4), in Buffer nerve denervated dogs, and in spinal dogs by Suresh (23), who concluded that the changes were due to some local mechanism. Angelicas (2), on the other hand, studied the effect of hypovolemia induced in dogs by ligating their venae cavae. Altschule et al (1) studied the effect of intravenous administration of fluids in men.

All these authors (1, 2, 4, 23) found the EKG changes to be quite variable, and observed an increase or decrease or sequentially both, in amplitude of various waves. Leaven (14) confirmed this variability of changes in the surface EKG, but he also noted that the results were more uniform on recording the potentials directly with endocardial and epicardial electrodes. What then, happens between the production of potentials by the myocardium, and their recording by the surface EKG?

EKG is a surface representation of electrical activity of cardiac dipole suspended in a volume conductor (thorax) which is, contrary to Einthoven's assumption, far from homogenous (Einthoven was aware of this, but he had practical reasons for the assumption). Intracardiac blood is 3-4 times as conductive of electricity as the myocardium, and the latter in turn, is about 10 times as conductive as the surrounding lungs (5).

The highly conductive intracavity blood short circuits the tangential dipoles and augments the radial ones, the so called

Brody effect (5). Increasing the conductivity of blood further by increasing the plasma volume, or by decreasing the red cell blood mass, or by overall hemodilution (9) will have greater effect.

The same can be achieved by increasing the end-diastolic volume (14). The effect theoretically predicted by Brody (5) was confirmed using model experiments by Nelson (17), while its converse was verified by Horan (10) by reducing the conductivity of blood by insufflation of cardiac ventricles of dogs with carbon dioxide.

In the present study, healthy individuals drank up to twelve glasses of water. This need not measurably increase the total plasma volume (13). Serum osmolality is known to decrease in patients with psychogenic polydipsia (11) and it may have decreased a little in this study. More likely is the increase in the end-diastolic volume to deliver the excess water to the kidneys. Although the data presented here do not allow one to sort out the relative importance of these factors, all these would have the additive effect on EKG.

Translation of theoretical predictions of Brody (5) and others into practical terms is complex, but these appear to be the best available possible explanations for our observations. Table: 2 is based on the works of Brody (5), Durrer (7), and Scher (18). The P wave dipoles are tangential to the atrial cavity, which can account for the flattening of the P wave (figure: 1) with forced water intake.

A q wave produced by septal depolarization, which is radial, is expected to be augmented (figure: 1), while the Q wave in aVR, produced also in part by right ventricular depolarization, may get smaller (figure: 2) as the latter is more tangential; for the same reason, a right ventricular R wave (Rs pattern) may get smaller (figure: 3). A left ventricular R wave (qR pattern) is radial and it may get bigger (figure: 1).

The S wave is a left ventricular wave produced by radial dipoles, and as predicted, it showed augmentation (figure: 4). A part of the S wave is produced by tangential dipoles, during the terminal part of the QRS (18). Therefore, some attenuation may have occurred but was not observed. The terminal s wave (qRs pattern) actually appeared for the first time with forced intake (figure: 3).

Lamb (12) discussed the effect of ventricular filling on QRS amplitude in $S_1S_2S_3$ conduction and suggested that the end diastolic volume may not affect the s wave which occurs so late, but the latter may become more prominent because of diminution of other left ventricular forces.

The production of T wave is very complex (24). In the present study, the T wave was flattened (figure: 1, 3) as if it was produced by tangential dipoles. Nelson (16) also observed a decrease in T wave magnitude with an increase in the conductivity of the blood. T wave flattening was also observed in the men who were given infusions (1) and in the newborns whose end-diastolic volume was increased (21).

Wilson (24) showed that flattening of T wave could be produced by drinking ice cold water. His subject was lying down supine and the changes were explained on the basis of cooling of the ventricles by *direct* contact with fundus of the stomach. In the present study, the subjects reclined at 45^0 angle and drank only cool water.

In addition to the conductivity of the intracardiac blood and ventricular volume (16), heart rate (12), and conductivity of the chest wall, which may change with hydration (22) are to be taken into account. An increase in the amplitude of some waves with a concurrent decrease in others, rules out the insulating effect of the chest wall water. The effect of respiration was avoided by taking the mean amplitude of the three largest QRS complexes.

There was no evidence of changes in the electrical axes or in position of the heart. Mutual cancellation of simultaneous vectors also complicated the matter. Caloric deprivation was present throughout, but the EKG changes were not progressive. Our data do not permit any comment on circadian rhythmicity of changes in the amplitude. T wave acrophase is known to occur in the afternoon (3), which was seen in one subject who did not show any flattening of the T wave (figure: 4).

Unlike the studies done in the experimental animals who were given massive transfusions (15), or were subjected to drastic volume depletion (2) with resultant severe hemodynamic disturbances, the present study demonstrates the variability of amplitude in healthy adult men and women who did not have any hemodynamic impairment. Thus, EKG voltage is affected by oral and parenteral intake, heart rate, ventricular volume, body build, changes in hematocrit, phases of respiration, etc. In the light of these, and the observations reported here, it seems that a fresh look at the voltage criteria for various diagnoses is in order.

Appreciating the sensitivity of amplitude to hydration may obviate unnecessary work up for low voltage to rule out the possibility of pericardial effusion, hypothyroidism, etc. Maybe, like fasting blood sugar, a fasting cardiogram (or under some other such standardization) should be obtained in euhydrated individuals, when voltage is an important consideration.

Changes in amplitude as a monitor of hydration is an interesting possibility, the practical application of which is curtailed by the variability of changes in different leads, generation of inconstant amount of current by different hearts, and the effect of diseases, viz., infarction, etc., on the amplitude of QRS. These changes in amplitude due to those in hydration can account for some day to day and other heretofore unexplained variations in the electrocardiograms.

In conclusion, data are presented to show that in healthy adult volunteers, amplitude of various EKG waves is affected by state of hydration, and (it is postulated that it) is attributable to the concomitant changes in the volume and the conductivity of the intracardiac blood.

Acknowledgements: The author thanks Dr. Sunil Amerasinghe for
technical support.

BIBLIOGRAPHY

1. Altschule MD, Gillian DR.
   The effects on the cardiovascular system of fluids administered
   intravenously in man.
   J. Clinical Investigation 1938, 17:401-411.
2. Angelicas ET, Gokhan N.
   Influence of venous inflow volume on the magnitude of the
   QRS potentials in vivo.
   Cardiology 1963, 42:337-348.
3. Alsatian NL, Adamtinan KG, Gregorian SV, Bagadassarian
   RA, Assertion DG.
   Circadian rhythms of ECG T-wave, arterial pressure and heart
   rate in patients with ischemic heart disease.
   Chronobiologia 19880, 7:481-492.
4. Bhatnagar NP, Gupta ML.
   Electrocardiographic changes during hypovolemia on dogs.
   Indian J Physiol and Pharmacy 1968, 12:71-74.
5. Brody DA.
   A theoretical analysis of intracavitary blood mass influence on
   the heart lead relationship.
   Circulation Research 1965, 4:731-738.
6. Comroe JH.
   Retrospectroscope. Insights into medical discovery.
   Von Gear Press, Menlo Park, California. 1977, p. 89-98.
7. Durrer D.
   The human heart. Aspects of its excitation.
   Transactions and studies of the College of Physicians of Phila-
   delphia, 1966 (fourth series) 33:159-170.
8. Hass HG, in
   Handbook of physiology, section 2, Circulation vol. I,

Hamilton WF, Philip D (Section editors),
Am Physiol Soc, Washington, DC. 1962, p. 323-415.

9. Kirsch FG, Texter EC jr, Wood LA, et al.
The electrical conductivity of blood.
Blood 1950, 5:1017-1035.

10. Horan LG, Andrea RL, Yoffee HF.
The effect of intracavitary carbon dioxide on surface potentials in the intact canine chest.
Am Heart J 1961, 61:504-514.

11. Kleemen CR, Vorherr H.
Water metabolism and the neurohypophysial hormones (in)
Duncan's Diseases of Metabolism
W. B. Saunders Company, Philadelphia, 1969, p. 1103-1149.

12. Lamb LE.
The effects of respiration on the electrocardiogram in relation to differences in right and left ventricular stroke volume.
Am Heart J 1957, 54:342-351.

13. Lawson, Hamden C, in
Handbook of Physiology, Section 2, Circulation Vol I.
Hamilton WF, Philip D (Section editors),
Am Physiol Soc, Washington, DC. 1962, p. 458.

14. Leaven J, Chatterjee K, Tiber JV, Parmley WW.
Reduction in ventricular endocardial and epicardial potentials during acute increments in left ventricular volume.
Am Heart J. 1979, 98:200-206.

15. Miller LW, Collins JA, Sherman L, Ladenson J.
Massive transfusion in swine.
Surgical Forum, 1977, 28:21-23.

16. Nelson CV, Chatterjee M, Angelicas ET, Hoechst HH.
Model studies on the effect of the intracardiac blood on the electrocardiogram.
Am Heart J, 1961, 62:83-92.

17. Nelson CV, Rand PW, Angelicas ET.

Effect of intracardiac blood on the spatial vecterocardiogram. Results in the dog.
Circulation Research 1972, 31:95-102.

18. Scher AM, Young AC.
Ventricular depolarization and the genesis of QRS.
Annals of NY Acad of Sciences, 1957, 65(6):768-778.

19. Shah BS.
Mirror-image relationship between body temperature and pulse rate.
JAMA, 1979, 242: p. 2760.

20. Shah BS.
A simplified extracorporeal approach to experimental ventilatory failure.
ASAIO Journal, 1985, 8:223-227.

21. Sossa ML, Rubio GG, Krater SK.
Influencia de la transfusion planetaria en el electrocardiogram del recline NiCad.
Arch Inst Cardiol Mex, 1973, 43:80-86.

22. Spence JA, Baliga R, Neighbor J, Septic J, Fleischmann I.
Changes during hemodialysis in total body water, cardiac output and chest fluid as detected by bioelectrical impedance analysis.
Trans Am Soc Artif Int Organs, 1979, 25:51-55.

23. Suresh TP.
Regression pattern of amplitude of electrocardiographic waves during intravenous infusion in intact, Buffer nerve denervated and spinal dogs.
Ibid. 1978, 22:249-262.

24. Wilson FN, Finch R.
The effects of drinking iced - water upon the form of the T deflection of the electrocardiogram.
Heart, 1923, 10:275-278.

32. INTERPLAY OF CIGARETTE SMOKING, DRUG ABUSE, SEASON OF BIRTH, AND POSTOPERATIVE COMPLICATIONS[31]

Bharat S. Shah, M.D.
Medical Specialist

Rogelio Foster, M.D.
Director of Medicine

ABSTRACT

Objective: To explore the relationship of postoperative complications with psychiatric and medical diagnoses, therapeutic interventions, and patient related factors.

Method: A retrospective records review study of psychiatric inpatients who had any surgery done during the 18 months ending on February 28, 2003, was performed. From the 55 patients record screened, 28 (19 men and 9 women, mean age 47 years) met the inclusion criterion of having an at least one inch long, surgically made or treated, visible wound. Data regarding their diagnoses, diet, and drug therapies, smoking habits, and surgical procedure(s) were collected. Two tailed Exact Probabilities were computed.

Results: Of the 28 patients, eight (29%) had developed one or more postoperative complications, viz., wound dehiscence (4), incisional hernia (2), seroma (3), etc. The African Americans (64% of the sample) had fewer (36%) complications (p = 0.09). All eight patients with complication(s) were from the group of 20 smokers (Fisher's One Tailed Exact p = 0.04). All wound problems occurred in patients

---

[31] From the Medical Services of Manhattan Psychiatric Center (affiliation of New York University Medical Center).

who had been born during spring and summer (Fisher's Two Tailed Exact p = 0.0005). Season of birth was a predictor of wound complications, independent of patients' smoking habits.

Conclusion: Postoperative wound complications are associated with patients' season of birth, smoking habits, and race. These findings strongly suggest the need for an aggressive approach to cigarette smoking by patients during the perioperative period; maybe, more so in case of those born during spring and summer.

Citation: *Shah BS.*
Interplay of cigarette smoking, drug abuse, season of birth, and postoperative complications. In Questions, Answers, and Exclamations from the Garage of a Clinical Researcher. P. 206 - 220, 2011 Setubandh Publications, New York.

Key Words: African Americans   Smoking
                   Season of birth   Complications

INTRODUCTION

Concurrent medical and surgical illnesses complicate the course of treatment of psychiatric conditions, and impose extra burden of physical and mental stress on patients. Treatments of most of these illnesses require transferring the patients to an acute care hospital, thereby interrupting his or her psychiatric care. Follow up clinic visits add personnel costs incurred for escorting the patient. Any adverse outcome of a surgical procedure aggravates all these by several magnitudes.

The Medical Services at our psychiatric facility reviewed outcomes of all surgical procedures during an 18 month period to determine the factor(s) that differentiate between patients with and without complications. The findings presented here are of practical importance, and they provide material for further research in an entirely new direction.

MATERIALS AND METHODS

This was a retrospective, non-interventional review of patients records, and gathering information from staff members who had cared for them in the peri-operative period. Records of all patients who had had any surgical procedure done to them between September 1, 2001, and February 28, 2003, (18 months) were screened.

These were scrutinized applying the sole inclusion criterion, viz. the presence of a surgically made or treated, at least one inch long, externally visible wound. That resulted in exclusion of endoscopic procedures, dental, ear-nose-throat interventions, vaginal gynecological surgery, minor traumatic lacerations not requiring suturing, and so on.

Procedures are done at one of the four hospitals where our patients are referred to. Patients go there for preoperative assessment, operation itself, and immediate postoperative care. Then they return to our hospital, and generally stay in a special area designated as Medical Infirmary, under very close observation, until they have recovered enough to return to their prior wards. Records from these hospitals were not reviewed, except for their discharge summaries, recommendations received from them, and consultants' notes received after follow up clinic visits.

Patients data included their name, race, sex, date of birth, hospital record number, and patients' ward. Clinical data included psychiatric and medical diagnoses, diet and drug therapies, and laboratory data, viz. complete blood count, chemistry (glucose, cholesterol, triglycerides, total proteins, albumin, globulin). Patients' height and weight are routinely recorded every month. Any gain or loss was computed. Peri-operative smoking habits were recorded by asking the care takers.

Details of operative procedures, viz. nature of intervention, description of the wound and its progress, and follow up care, were recorded. An adverse outcome or complication was defined as any of the following:

1. Wound dehiscence, wherein the wound opened up partly or completely, revealing the raw, non-healing tissues.

2. Wound infection, which manifested as fever > 101°F, purulent discharge, or redness around the surgical site persisting for more than a week.

3. Seroma formation or collection of more than 100 ml serous fluid at the operative site, requiring aspiration or open surgical drainage.

4. Incisional hernia, indicating weakness and an opening underneath the superficially healed scar.

Presence or absence of complication(s) was then correlated with that of various diagnostic, therapeutic, and patient related factors using 2 x 2 tables. Since some cells in these tables had a "zero" value in them, Fisher's Exact One-tailed or Two-tailed Probabilities computed for statistical significance.

OBSERVATIONS AND RESULTS

Initial screening revealed 55 patients who had had some surgery during the 18 month period. Of these, 28 patients met the sole inclusion criterion. There were 18 African Americans, eight Hispanics, and two whites. There were 19 men, and 9 women. Their mean age was 47 years.

One Hispanic woman, included in these 28 patients had two unrelated operations during that period, and therefore, is counted as two distinct patients. Since one intervention in her case was uneventful, and the other was complicated, most of her data canceled or balanced themselves out. As an important footnote, her uneventful procedure was the only instance of any patient receiving a nicotine replacement and buspirone treatment in the peri-operative period.

With some overlap patients' psychiatric diagnoses included schizophrenia (20), bipolar disorder (4), depression (2), and personality disorder (5). A history of substance abuse was present in 19 patients. Medical diagnoses were, hypertension (9), positive tuberculin skin test (9), bronchial asthma (6), obesity, that is, BMI > 30 (5), hyperlipidemia (5), Human Immune Deficiency Virus infection (3), epilepsy (2), diabetes mellitus (2), hypothyroidism (1), and hepatitis: C infection (1).

Our patients were treated at one of the four referral hospitals in New York City. They treated 23, 3, 1, and 1 patients, and from these patients, 7 (30.0% rate for that facility, 87% of all complications), 1 (33.3% rate, 13% of the total), occurred in the first two hospitals.

Procedures	(#)	Complications	(#)
Open cholecystectomy	3	Wound dehiscence	1
		Incisional hernia	1
		Seroma aspiration/ drainage	1
Open reduction of hip fracture	2		
Inguinal herniorrhaphy	2		

Suturing of head laceration	2		
Excision of lipoma	2	Seroma aspiration/drainage	1
Hydrocoelectomy	2	Seroma aspiration/drainage	1
		Hematocoele	1
Pancreatic cysto-jejuno-stomy	1	Incisional hernia repair	1
		Seroma aspiration/drainage	1
Caesarian Section	1		
Abdominal subtotal hysterectomy	1	Wound dehiscence	1
Radical hysterectomy, bilateral salpingo-oophorectomy	1		
Ovarian cystectomy	1		
Thoracotony for lung cancer	1		
Nephrolithotomy	1		
Wrist tumor excision	1		
Internal fixation of hand fracture	1		
Repair of a hemodialysis shunt	1		

Pilonidal cyst excision	1	Infection	1
		"Z-plasty" re-pair	1
Excision biopsy of			
Breast mass	1		
Testicular mass	1		
Lymph node	1		
Perianal polyp	1		
TOTAL	28		12

Some patients had more than complication. Eight patients had developed 12 complications. None had developed pulmonary or systemic infection. All patients eventually recovered completely. There was no mortality attributable to any of the complications. Compared to the whites, and the Hispanics, the African Americans (64% of the total) had a tendency to develop fewer (36%) complications (Exact One tailed p =0.07, Two tailed p = 0.09).

Occurrence of complications was not associated with any of the psychiatric diagnosis, dietary or pharmacotherapy. Similarly, it showed no association with any medical condition, including hypertension, diabetes mellitus, obesity, HIV infection, or any medical drug therapy. No patient had significant anemia or hypoproteinemia.

Complications and Smoking:

Of the 28 patients, 20 (71%) smoked >5 cigarettes daily. Our hospital does not provide free cigarettes, but has five smoking periods of 15 minutes each, set aside every day for restricted and supervised smoking by patients. Staff is not permitted to smoke.

These 20 patients took all such breaks, smoked more than one cigarette during some breaks, or asked for additional cigarettes between breaks, or got agitated at times, when their request was not fulfilled. They constituted the Heavy Smokers group. All 12 complications occurred in this group (risk rate for a heavy smoker to develop a complication: 0.4, Odds 0.66, or a 66% likelihood).

From the remaining eight patients, the Non-or Nominal Smokers group, seven were nonsmokers (25% of the total 28), and one patient smoked up to five cigarettes a day. That patient did not always smoke during every break. Nor did he demand to smoke more than one cigarette during a break, and he never got agitated when denied a cigarette. Not a single postoperative complication occurred in this group. Thus, the Odds Ratio for heavy smokers, as compared to nonsmokers or nominal smokers to develop complications was infinity.

Since our main interest was in the peri-operative smoking habits, rather than going by the usual pack years of smoking history, we opted for the above behavioral criteria, to accommodate the observer variability without sacrificing accuracy. Difference between the two groups was statistically significant (Fisher's One Tailed Exact $p = 0.04$). The hospital has become a smoke free facility since July 24, 2003.

Complications and the Season of Birth:

None of the complications occurred in patients who were born during the fall and winter (9/21-3/20). All twelve complications occurred in the patients who were born in spring or summer (3/21-9/20). The risk for the latter group to develop a complication was 0.53, Odds 1.14, and the Odds Ratio between the two groups was infinity. These results were statistically significant (Two Tailed Exact $p = 0.0005$). Season of birth showed no association with the diagnosis of schizophrenia, or with smoking habit. It was not a proxy or surrogate variable.

Seasonality of Birth and Past Drug Abuse:

The seasonality of birth did show a significant association with a history of substance abuse, i.e., the latter was more common in patients (Risk Ratio 1.81, Odds Ratio 5.5) born during spring and summer (One Tailed Exact p = 0.04, Two Tailed p = 0.05). A history of substance abuse was not associated with complications at all. Nor did it show any relation with smoking.

DISCUSSION

Surgical procedures are stressful events even for those not suffering from a mental disease, but are more so in psychiatric patients. Any adverse outcome of surgery is understandably, doubly distressing. Our patients are referred to four of the several hospitals in New York City. The data presented do not allow us to compare the care provided by those hospitals.

Impaired wound healing is known to be caused by diseases like diabetes mellitus, poor nutrition, drugs like steroids and non-steroidal anti-inflammatory agents-NSAIDs (1,2), immuno-suppression (3), etc., a few of which were present in our patients, but only in isolated instances, and were not associated with any complications.

Wound dehiscence is an uncommon (4) complication, occurring in less than 1% of cases, but carrying 20% mortality. Common known causes of dehiscence are infection, imperfect technique, and increased intra-abdominal pressure. In a large study of 89 instances of dehiscence occurring in 19206 major abdominal operations, Pavlidis et al (5) found age > 65 years, emergency operation, cancer, ascites, obesity, and steroids to be important causes, and sex, diabetes, anemia, and pulmonary disease to be unimportant causes of dehiscence.

Complications and Smoking:

Smoking is not specifically mentioned as a cause of dehiscence in the literature reviewed. The present data showed a strong link between the severity of cigarette smoking and occurrence of postoperative complications. Smoking has been shown to affect adversely, wound healing after breast cancer surgery (6), and that on the hand wherein cessation of smoking led to resumption of wound healing (7). Besides inhibiting the necessary growth factors, smoking also prevents deposition of collagen (8), and lowers the local tissue oxygen tension (9).

All three of these ingredients are crucial for proper wound healing. Lowering of oxygen tension in tissues is mediated through adrenergic vasoconstriction and through formation of carbon monoxide hemoglobin, which does not readily release oxygen to the tissues, because of much higher affinity of the carboxyhemoglobin for oxygen.

There is an extensive body of literature showing that cigarette smoking is one of the most prevalent, preventable cause of morbidity and mortality in the general population. Campaigns for cessation of smoking have successfully decreased the prevalence of smoking in the U.S. adult population to 24%. At the same time, prevalence of smoking in psychiatric facilities has remained 2-3 times as high. In this study, unchanged from a previous one (10) in the same institution, 75% of patients in our hospital were smokers.

Smoking and its cessation in psychiatric hospitals is a complex and thorny issue, generating lot of heat and smoke, literally and figuratively. In the not so remote past, cigarettes were used as pacifiers to keep patients with unmanageable behavior problems under control. Now, several psychiatric facilities have successfully gone smoke-free, generally without any of the predicted dire consequences (11).

Success rates of smoking cessation programs for mental patients are similar to those achieved in nonpsychiatric populations (12). Smoking may apparently alleviate some symptoms of schizophrenia, either directly or indirectly by counteracting some side effects of psychotropic drugs by accelerating their metabolism, thereby lowering their blood levels and hence, their effectiveness (13). In the genetically predisposed individuals, it may alter the metabolic pathway, and in turn, lead to production of toxic metabolites (14).

Therefore, it is imperative that even psychiatric patients be counseled and helped in every possible way to make them refrain from smoking, at least, in the perioperative period. If that cannot be done, if at all feasible, one should seriously consider postponing or canceling all elective procedures in heavy smokers with a 66% likelihood of complications. Maybe, that's what *primum non nocere* (First, do no harm) is all about.

A retrospective study like the present one cannot establish causation, but has to limit itself to establishing associations. The study sample is narrowly selected, therefore, its results cannot be simply extrapolated to the general population. Also, some questions like, "Why did we not see so many complications in the past, when smoking was more freely accessible in mental hospitals?" cannot be answered, and have to be left for other studies.

Complications and Season of Birth:

The association of complications with being born in the middle half of the year, several times stronger than the one with smoking, is fascinating and puzzling at the same time. Patients with schizophrenia are more likely to be born during the northern hemispheric winter (15), and the theory of a viral infection (16) occurring during that period or nine months earlier has been proposed as one of the explanations.

Since seasonality of birth of patients with schizophrenia (winter) is quite different from that of those with surgical complications (spring and summer), one wonders whether schizophrenia has a protective effect against postoperative complications. Our data do not provide answer to this interesting hypothesis. In our sample, patients with schizophrenia did not show any seasonality of birth, nor did they show any association with smoking. Our patients census of the entire hospital (unpublished personal data from 706 patients, 1998) did show seasonality of winter birth in patients with schizophrenia.

Seasonality of Birth and Past Drug Abuse:

The mid year seasonality of birth showed a striking association (statistical significance, Exact p = 0.04 one tailed, and 0.05 two tailed) with a history of substance abuse. The latter was 5.5 times more likely (Odds Ratio) in those who were born between March 21 and September 20. Our findings are in sharp contrast to those of Goldberg et al (17), who found patients with substance abuse to be more likely to have been born during the fall. Theirs was a large national study, unlike the present very small sample limited to psychiatric patients with surgical procedures.

Seasonality of birth of patients with a history of substance abuse also raises a possibility of a peri-natal or peri-conception viral infection, and other factor(s), leading up to an addictive personality. Lot more work is needed before this can be settled.

Although the seasonality of births showed a relationship with complications, as did smoking, the former is not a surrogate variable for smoking, i.e., there was no interrelationship between the two. On the other hand, association of seasonality with a history of substance abuse showed no association either with surgical complications, or with smoking. Much larger samples are needed to determine the importance, if any, of these newly observed phenomena.

In conclusion, retrospective data are presented showing that postoperative complications are associated with season of birth, peri-operative smoking habit, and to some extent, with belonging to the white or the Hispanic race. Similar seasonality of births, but unrelated to complications, was observed in those with past drug abuse.

BIBLIOGRAPHY

1.   Karukonda RK, Flynn TC, Boh EE, McBurney EI, Russo GG, and Millikan LE.
     The Effects of drugs on wound healing: part I.
     International J of Dermat. 2009; 39:250-257.

2.   Karukonda RK, Flynn TC, Boh EE, McBurney EI, Russo GG, and Millikan LE.
     The Effects of drugs on wound healing: part II. Specific classes of drugs and their effect on healing of wounds.
     International J of Dermat. 2009; 39:321-333.

3.   Scaffer MR, Fuchs N, Proksch B, Bongartz M, Beiter T, and Becker HD.
     Tacrolimus impairs wound healing: a possible role of de-creased nitric oxide synthesis.
     Transplantation; 65(6):813-818.

4.   Moosa AR, Jones ML, Scott M. in
     Savitson DC, Editor
     Textbook of Surgery, Philadelphia, PA.
     W. B. Saunders & Co. 1986;331-345.

5.   Pavlidis TE, Gelatianos IN, Papaziogas BT, Lazaridis CN, Atmatzidis KS, Makris JG, Papaziogas TB,
     Complete dehiscence of the abdominal wound and incrimi-nating factors.
     Eur J Surg 2001;167(5):351-354.

6.   Sorenson LT, Horby J, Friis E, Pilsgaard B, Jorgensen T,
     Smoking as a risk factor for wound healing and infection in breast cancer surgery.
     Eur J Surg Oncol 2002;28(2):815-820.

7.   Mosely LH, Finseth F,
     Cigarette smoking: Impairment of digital blood flow and wound healing in hand.

Hand 1977;9(2):97-101.

8. Jorgensen KN, Kallehave F, Christiansen E, Siana JE, Gottrub F.
    Less collagen production in smokers.
    Surgery 1998;123(4):450-455.

9. Jensen JA, Goodson MD, Hopf HW, Hunt TK.
    Cigarette smoking decreases tissue oxygen.
    Arch Surg 1991; 126:1131-1134.

10. Shah BS, Ratner H.
    Anti-convulsant drugs, smoking, and body weights in psychiatric inpatients.
    NY State J Med 1993;93:16-17.

11. El-Gubaly N, Cathcart J, Currie S, Brown D, Gloster S.
    Public health and therapeutic aspects of smoking bans in mental health and addiction settings.
    Psych Serv 2002'53(12):1617-1622.

12. Jorm AF, Rodgers B, Jacomb PA, Christensen H, Henerson S, and Korten AF.
    Smoking and mental health:
    Results from a community survey.
    Med J Australia 1999;170(2):74-77.

13. Haustein KO, Haffner S, Woodcock BG.
    A review of pharmacological aspects of smoking cessation in psychiatric patients.
    Int J Clin Pharmacol Ther 2002; 40(9):404-418.

14. Seppala NH, Leinonen ML, Kivisto KT.
    Clozapine serum concentrations are lower in smoking than in non-smoking schizophrenic patients.
    Pharmacol Toxicol 1999; 85(5):244-246.

15. Torrey EF, Rawlings RR, Ennis JM, Merrill DD, and Flores DS.

    Birth seasonality in the bipolar disorder, schizophrenia, schizoaffective disorder, and stillbirths.

    Schizophr Res 1996;18(2):141-149.

16. Takei N, Mortensen PB, Klaening U, Murray RM, Sham PC, O'Calaghan E, Munk-Jorgensen P.

    Relationship between in utero exposure to influenza epidemics and risk of schizophrenia in Denmark.

    Biol Psychiatry 1996;40(9):817-824.

17. Goldberg AE, Newlin DB.

    Season of birth and substance abuse: findings from a large national sample.

    Alcohol Clin Exp Res 2000; 24(6):774-780.

33. PHENYTOIN, CALCIUM CHANNEL BLOCKING AGENTS, AND HIV INFECTION[32]

Bharat S. Shah, M.D.
Asst. Director of Medicine

Adnan M. Khdair, M.D.
Research Fellow

ABSTRACT

Background: Phenytoin is reported to prevent the human immune deficiency virus (HIV) infection of T4 lymphocytes in the tissue cultures, possibly by preventing a rise in intracellular calcium level.

Objectives: To test the hypothesis that treatment with phenytoin and calcium channel blocking agents, prescribed for unrelated reasons, will be associated a lower likelihood of having a positive test for HIV infection.

Design: A noninvasive, retrospective, data-review study.

Setting: An inner city hospital in New York City.

Methods: The test group consisted of 53 patients who were known to have been tested for the HIV infection, out of 850 patients (1350 prescriptions), and were receiving phenytoin, isradipine, nifedipine, diltiazem, and/or verapamil. The control group consisted of 53 patients, individually matched for race, sex, and age, but who were not receiving any of the drugs mentioned, and were also known to have been tested for the HIV infection.

---

[32] From: Dept. of Medicine
   Woodhull Medical and Mental Health Center
   760 Broadway, Brooklyn, NY. 11206.

Interventions: No intervention regarding HIV testing or drug therapy was done.

Results and

Conclusions: Phenytoin and isradipine were 2.5 and 3.0 times more likely (McNemar's Test) to be associated with a negative test for HIV infection. Nifedipine, diltiazem, and verapamil showed no such association. The results were statistically significant at fisher's Exact Two Tailed p = 0.025.

Citation: *Shah BS.*

                Phenytoin, calcium channel blocking agents, and HIV infection. In

                Questions, Answers, and Exclamations from the Garage of a Clinical Researcher. P. 221 - 228, 2011 Setubandh Publications, New York.

Key Words: Seizures   Toxoplasmosis

                    Hypertension   Cryptococcal Meningitis

INTRODUCTION

It was reported in 1986 that T4 human lymphocytes treated with phenytoin *in vitro* (1) and *in vivo* (1) were able to resist the infection with human immune deficiency virus (HIV), probably by preventing the rise in the intracellular calcium (2). We did a study to see whether therapy with phenytoin and calcium channel blocking drugs is associated a decreased likelihood of HIV seroconversion.

We present the data from a retrospective, observational study that raises the possibility of employing phenytoin (PHT) and some calcium channel blocking agents (CCBs) that are already being commonly prescribed for other indications, to protect the T4 lymphocytes during the early stages of the HIV infection, or even prevent the infection of these cells altogether.

MATERIALS AND METHODS

Woodhull Medical and Mental Health Center is an inner city hospital in Brooklyn, New York, and is operated by the New York City Health and Hospitals Corporation. Its catchment area houses predominantly black and Hispanic communities. It serves a large number of patients with HIV infection, related mainly to intravenous drug abuse and to multiple sexual partners. There is a very small proportion of homosexuals. All the HIV counseling and testing is conducted by its AIDS (Acquired Immune Deficiency Syndrome) program.

Our study was a retrospective, non-experimental one, based on existing data from the AIDS program, the hospital pharmacy, and the Medical Records department. We obtained copies of all prescriptions issued to adult patients during a two months period, for phenytoin and/or the CCBs, viz. Isradipine[33], nifedipine, diltiazem, and verapamil. These patients were cross checked with the database of the AIDS program to identify those who had been tested for seroconversion for HIV (test group). No drug therapy, or HIV testing was prescribed or otherwise encouraged just for this study.

Those patients on phenytoin therapy, whose records indicated that the therapy was instituted to treat the seizures caused by AIDS related cerebral toxoplasmosis or cryptococcal meningitis, were excluded. Far advanced AIDS per se, or noncompliance with therapy was not a criterion for exclusion.

From the AIDS program database, we found a control group of same number of patients who were individually matched for age, race, and sex, who were also known to have had been tested for HIV seroconversion, but who were not receiving any of the five medications mentioned earlier. During the matching, re-

---

[33] Isradipine (Dynacirc) is no longer marketed in the US.

sults of the HIV test were blanked out on the computer screen to avoid bias, and were looked up subsequently.

Both groups were stratified according to the drug therapy that the test group had received. Each individually matched pair of patients was then examined using the McNemar's Chi-Square test for the factor "freedom from the HIV infection," i.e., for the HIV test (-), and Odds Ratios were computed. Fisher's Exact Two Tailed Probability was calculated for comparing phenytoin-isradipine with the rest of the drugs.

OBSERVATIONS AND RESULTS

The data are presented in the accompanying table. Initially, we were able to obtain 1350 prescriptions, issued to 850 patients. Of these, 53 patients were found to have been tested for the HIV seroconversion. Two patients were getting two drugs each. One was on phenytoin plus nifedipine, while the other was on phenytoin plus diltiazem. Both of these patients appear under phenytoin, as well as the other drugs in the table (row A).

There were two patients who were on phenytoin, who met the pre-established exclusion criteria, and were deleted from the row C, under phenytoin, in the table. One of them had cryptococcal meningitis, while the other had cerebral toxoplasmosis. Both patients were being treated with phenytoin for the first time for the seizures induced by these AIDS related conditions. Excluding these two patients canceled out the two extra entries mentioned above, to keep the total at 53 pairs.

As shown in the table (row D), there were two pairs in which both members were HIV (+). There was only one patient on verapamil who, like the control, was negative for HIV (row A). Three patients on nifedipine and one on diltiazem were positive for HIV, while their respective controls were negative (row C). Phenytoin treatment was 2.5 times, and isradipine was 3 times more likely to be associated with a negative test for HIV.

HIV TEST		ISD	PHT	DLT	NFD	VRP	TOTAL
TEST	CNTRL						
A. —	—	5	16	2	12	1	36
B. —	+	3	5	0	0	0	8
C. +	—	1	2	1	3	0	7
D. +	+	1	1	0	0	0	2
Total:		10	24	3	15	1	53
Odds Ratio (B/C):		3.0	2.5	0/1	0/3	0/0	

Table: The table shows distribution of patients pairs according to the drug therapy, and into the rows A through D for McNemar's Chi-Square test. As an example, (row C) in seven pairs, the test patients had a positive test for HIV conversion, while the control patient had a negative one. ISD: isradipine, PHT: phenytoin, DLT: diltiazem, NFD: nifedipine, and VRP: verapimil.

If no exclusion criteria were applied, the Odds Ratio for phenytoin would have been 5/4 or 1.25, still a 25% more likelihood for being HIV negative. The difference in phenytoin-isradipine against the rest of the drugs was significant at $p = 0.025$ (Fisher's Two Tailed Exact).

DISCUSSION

At present there is no effective therapy[34] for prevention or treatment of adult HIV infection. Phenytoin was shown to prevent HIV infection of T4 cells in tissue culture when the drug was added in vitro or when it was given orally in therapeutic doses (1) to volunteers from whom the T4 cells were obtained. Phenytoin was able to prevent the primary infection, as well as the re-infection by the virus emerging from the destroyed T4 cells.

---

[34] This was written in early 1990s.

There was one clinical study which demonstrated the inability of phenytoin to alter the course of far advanced AIDS (3). This is not surprising, because phenytoin is not an anti-viral agent in the usual sense, but it apparently protects the T4 cells against the HIV. Cloyd (2) investigated the mechanism by which phenytoin protects the T4 cells, and found that it prevented the rise in intracellular calcium which heralds the HIV infection and the imminent death of that cell.

Our data suggest the possibility that phenytoin—which is also a calcium channel blocking agent (4) when used in therapeutic doses—and other such drugs can modulate, and maybe, prevent the HIV infection, especially in its early stages. The Odds Ratios of 2.5 (phenytoin) and 3.0 (isradipine) in favor of being HIV negative seem quite promising. These results need to be duplicated and to be furthered with prospective studies.

Lipton (5) while studying the CCBs for their possible protective effects against HIV-induced neuronal injury, found that diltiazem was ineffective, whereas verapamil was possibly effective in subtoxic concentrations. Our data agree regarding diltiazem, but we cannot comment on verapamil.

Dihydropyridine CCBs like nifedipine and nimodipine were (5) quite effective. Our study did not include any patient on nimodipine. However, our data regarding nifedipine are in stark contrast. Isradipine, also a dihydropyridine CCB which Lipton (5) did not study, showed the best results in our study, without requiring any help from exclusion criteria. Our data probably reflect the action of drugs on T4 lymphocytes, while Lipton's data deal with that on neurons. Selectivity of calcium channels to different CCBs varies from one cell type to another.

The comparison groups were matched for age, race, and sex, but not for the risk factors leading to the HIV infection. We did not interview the patients and the available information regarding the risk factors was not adequate. Nonetheless, it should be emphasized that all patients included in the study had been considered either by themselves or by others to be at risk for developing the HIV infection, and were sufficiently convinced of the necessity of being tested to consent for the same.

These results, although statistically significant, are still tentative and they suggest further course of action. One should refrain from raising one's hopes high. There is no reason yet to start prescribing phenytoin or isradipine to potentially or actually HIV (+) people, because it is hard to predict who will sero-convert and who would not. Cloyd's data (2) did show that phenytoin at times even favored the entry of the virus into the T4 cells. However, phenytoin is not considered to be contraindicated in the treatment of AIDS-related seizures, quite opposite is the case. Our data did not show any harm either, associated with phenytoin therapy for epileptic seizures in these patients, rather, the therapy may be beneficial.

In comparison to phenytoin and isradipine, nifedipine and diltiazem were associated with a (statistically significant at p = 0.025) five to ten fold likelihood of being associated with a positive test for HIV. Our study was designed to look for possible protection, rather than a predisposition. Some patients may have been already HIV positive when they were started on these drugs, Our data do not justify recommending to stop prescribing these two useful drugs.

In conclusion, we have presented the data of a retrospective study to suggest that phenytoin and isradipine are two and half to three times likely to be associated with a negative test for the HIV seroconversion.

BIBLIOGRAPHY

1.   Zimmer JP, Lehr HA, Kornhuber ME, Breitig D, Montagnier L, Gietzen K.
   Diphenylhydantoin (DPH) blocks HIV - receptor on T - lymphocyte surface
   Blut 1986; 53:447-450.

2.   Cloyd MW, Lynn WS, Ramsey K, Baron S.
   Inhibition of immunodeficiency virus (HIV - 1) infection by diphenylhydantoin (Dilantin) implicates role of cellular calcium in virus life cycle.
   Virology 1989; 173: 581-590.

3.   Kern W, Pecker U, Petzoldt D, Rasche H, Turowsky - Burwinkel G, Heimpel H, Vanck E.
   Treatment of symptomatic HIV infection with oral diphenylhydantoin.
   AIDS - Forscung (AIFO) 1988; 6:334.

4.   Shin-ichi I, Yamamoto N, Nomoto K, Sasaki K, Onodera K.
   Selective killing of human T cell lymphocytropic virus type I -transformed cell lines by a Damavaricin Fc derivative.
   J Antibiot 1989; 42:779-782.

5.   Lipton SA.
   Calcium channel antagonists and human immuno deficiency virus coat protein-mediated neuronal injury.
   Ann Neurol 1991; 30: 110-114.

34. REVISITING
THE CHOLESTEROL-VIOLENCE CONTROVERSY
WITH NEW OBSERVATIONS ON LIPID FRACTIONS:
A RETROSPECTIVE STUDY[35]

Bharat S. Shah, M.D.
Medical Specialist

ABSTRACT

Objectives: To explore the relationship, if any, of various lipid fractions with assaultive behavior in psychiatric inpatients, and to define the rationale of lipid lowering treatments in potentially and actually violent patients.

Design: Inpatient records of all "assaults" occurring during the five months ending on May 31, 2003, revealed 23 aggressors. A control group of 23 psychiatric patients, matched for age, sex, and inpatient location was selected. Records were reviewed for diagnoses, therapies, and total cholesterol, triglycerides, HDL-cholesterol (HDL-C), and LDL-cholesterol (LDL-C). Differences in the mean levels of these between the groups were compared for statistical significance.

Results: The mean total cholesterol level did not differ between the groups. The aggressors had a significantly higher mean level of triglycerides, a lower level of HDL-C, and a lower level of LDL-C corrected for BMI and HDL-C. These relationships persisted after being adjusted for mutual correlations of variables, lipid raising/lowering treatments, and confounding variables like the Body Mass Index (BMI).

---

[35] From the Medical Services of Manhattan Psychiatric Center (Affiliation of New York University Medical Center) Wards Island, New York, NY 10035.

Conclusions: Physically assaultive behavior in psychiatric inpatients is significantly associated with high triglycerides, low HDL-C, and low LDL-C fractions, but not with total cholesterol level. The data showed no contraindication to giving judicious cardiac prophylaxis to psychiatric patients by normalizing their lipid levels.

Limitations: More data are needed before conclusions of this retrospective study with a small sample of psychiatric inpatients can be applied to population at large.

Citation: *Shah BS.*

Revisiting the cholesterol-violence controversy with new observations on various lipid fractions: A retrospective study. In

Questions, Answers, and Exclamations from the Garage of a Clinical Researcher. P. 229 - 243, 2011 Setubandh Publications, New York.

Key Words:
Aggression   Atypical psychotropics
Hypolipidemic drugs   Low fat diet
Diabetes mellitus   Thyroid disease

INTRODUCTION

An association between low cholesterol level and violence was suggested by the Scandinavian study (1) which showed a decrease in cardiovascular mortality after lowering the total serum cholesterol level, offset by an increase in deaths attributed to violent causes. other studies reported a reduction in both, cardiovascular and overall mortality with lipid lowering drug therapy (2). Consequent to the ongoing controversy, the prudence of treating hyperlipidemia for prevention of cardiovascular events, and strokes (3) has been questioned. Use of the statin group of drugs to treat hyperlipidemia is reportedly not associated with an increase in violent deaths (4). Randomized controlled studies of statin group of drugs are being done (5).

On the other hand, according to some, there seems to be little or no controversy over the association of low total cholesterol with violence, physically assaultive behavior, and suicides in psychiatric patients (6), although some studies showed no such relationship (7). Most studies report only on total cholesterol and triglyceride levels, while data on other lipid fractions, viz., HDL-C (HDL Cholesterol), and LDL-C (LDL Cholesterol) are generally not available. Therefore, it is difficult to see whether an increase or a decrease, in which lipid fraction, is or is not associated with violence. The present study attempts to define the issue in terms of various lipid fractions in psychiatric patients.

The issue of treating potentially or actually violent psychiatric patients to lower their lipids for primary cardiac prevention raises an ethical concern: Does preventing cardiac death or stroke justify endangering the life of the patient and or of others? The data presented here provide a new perspective and it is hoped, a resolution of the dilemma.

MATERIALS AND METHODS

Manhattan Psychiatric Center is a 350 bed, inpatient psychiatric hospital in New York city, receiving many of its patients from the correctional (prison) system, and forensic facilities. A history of drug abuse, thefts, robbery, assaults, fights, suicide attempts, and homicide can be seen in many patients' records, some of these also occurring during the hospital stay.

The present study is a retrospective chart review, approved by the Institutional Review Board. Besides keeping records of medication errors, accidents, etc., the hospital maintains those of all violent incidents, e.g., fights, assaults, rapes, suicides, etc. Records of patients involved in incidents classified as "assaults" during the first five months of the year 2003 were reviewed. Aggressors were clearly identified in the reports.

Another group comprising of patients matched with the aggressors by age, sex, and the inpatient ward where they stayed, was selected as the control group. Patients from the latter group were not involved in any incident during the five month period. Lipids are affected by age, while the frequency and severity of violence differ in men and women. Therefore, the groups were matched for age and sex. Groups were compared for their medical and psychiatric diagnoses and lipid lowering or raising treatments with "atypical" psychotropic drugs like clozaril and olazapine (8).

All patients had lab results of total cholesterol and serum triglycerides levels in their records. Many of them had a complete lipid profile including total cholesterol, triglycerides, HDL-C, and LDL-C levels. If several test results were available, the one closest to the date of the incident was used for the study. No tests, diets, or drug therapies were ordered specifically for the study.

Data were checked and adjusted for effects of confounding variables, viz., lipid raising drugs (atypical psychotropics like olanzapine, clozaril, risperidal, ziprazidone, quetiapine), lipid lowering therapies like low fat diet, atorvastatin, pravastatin, and levothyroxine given to treat hypothyroidism. Since the study was centered mainly on lipid levels, no matter how achieved, no data on any patient receiving any of the above drugs were discarded, but were factored in the analysis.

Total cholesterol, HDL-C, LDL-C, and triglycerides were plotted and checked for their mutual correlations (Least Square method), and data were adjusted accordingly. They were also adjusted for confounding variables, e.g., the BMI (Body Mass

Index), computed for each patient using the formula BMI = body weight in kg/height in meters squared.

Levels of these lipid variables in aggressors and in controls were plotted and the difference in their mean values between groups was assessed for statistical significance using the "Student"-t test, and two tailed Exact Probabilities were computed.

OBSERVATIONS AND RESULTS

During the period January 1, through May 31, 2003, there were 44 incidents categorized as "assaults," wherein aggressors were clearly identified. There were 23 aggressors on whom complete records were available (out of 25). Six of these 23 patients were involved in multiple assaults (2-5 each). The control group of 23 patients was matched for age, sex, and inpatient location.

Each group included two women. Men were 24-62 years old. The groups did not differ significantly in their BMI, mean value for the aggressors was 34.32, that for the controls was 30.63, two-tailed $p = 0.08$.

Main psychiatric diagnoses included schizophrenia, bipolar disorder, personality disorder, drug abuse, and depression. Medical diagnoses included hypertension, diabetes mellitus (insulin dependent type I, and non-insulin dependent type II), obesity, hyperlipidemia, hypothyroidism, and seizures.

All 46 patients' records contained results of laboratory tests of total cholesterol and serum triglycerides levels. Out of 46 patients, 19 of them (seven aggressors, and 12 controls) had a complete lipid profile including total cholesterol, serum triglycerides, HDL-C, and LDL-C levels. Their mutual relationship and those with aggressors and control groups are presented below.

***

Mutual Correlations and Regressions of Variables:

1. HDL-C varied inversely linearly with the triglycerides level (y = 61.81 - 0.13x, R = -0.777, R-squared = 0.60, N = 19, p =0.0001).
2. HDL-C varied inversely with BMI (y = 69.11 - 0.90x, r = -0.503, R-squared = 0.25, N = 19, p = 0.028).

Difference in Lipid Fractions between Groups:

1. Total cholesterol showed no difference in the mean level between groups (figure: 1).

Figure: 1
Total Cholesterol Level

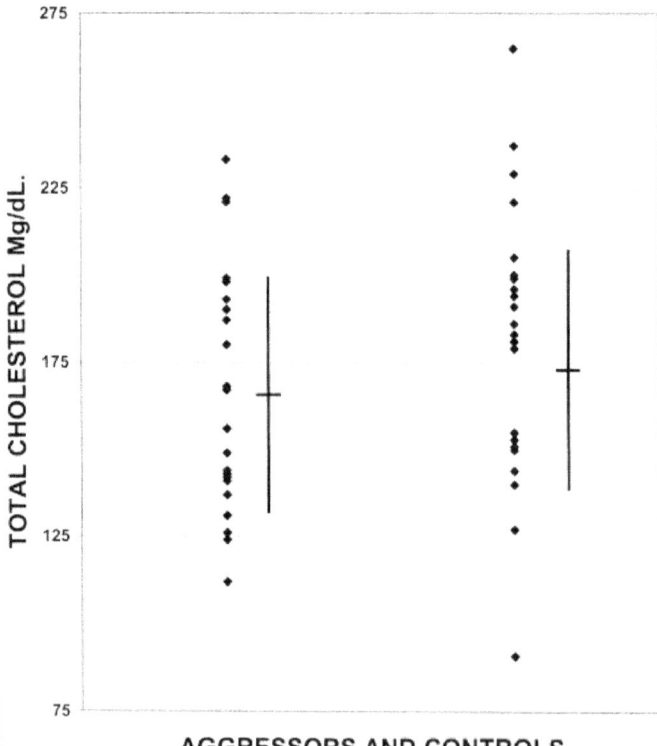

Figure: 1. Total cholesterol level did not differ significantly between groups. The mean levels ± one standard deviation are shown for aggressors and for controls (N = 46, not sta -tistically significantly significant, p > 0.05).

2. Serum triglycerides level (figure: 2) showed a higher mean level in the aggressors as compared the controls (p = 0.017). Adjusting for the BMI by keeping the latter constant at 20-30 did not affect the results (not shown), which remained significant at two tailed p = 0.03.

Figure: 2
Triglycerides Level of Groups

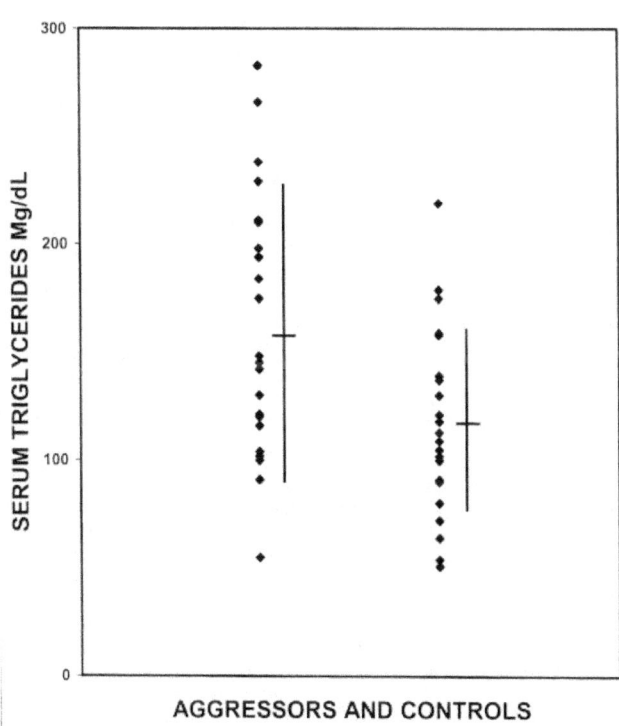

AGGRESSORS AND CONTROLS

Figure: 2. Difference in the mean serum tri-glycerides levels between aggressors and controls. Respective mean values ± one standard deviation are shown. Results were significant at p = 0.017, and they remained so after data were adjusted for the BMI, HDL-C, and use of atypical psychotropic drugs (not shown).

3. HDL-C level (figure: 3) showed a lower mean level in aggressors (p = 0.0001). Keeping BMI constant at 25-30 did not affect the relation of HDL-C within the groups, which still remained significant at two tailed p = 0.002.

Figure: 3
HDL-Cholesterol Level of Groups

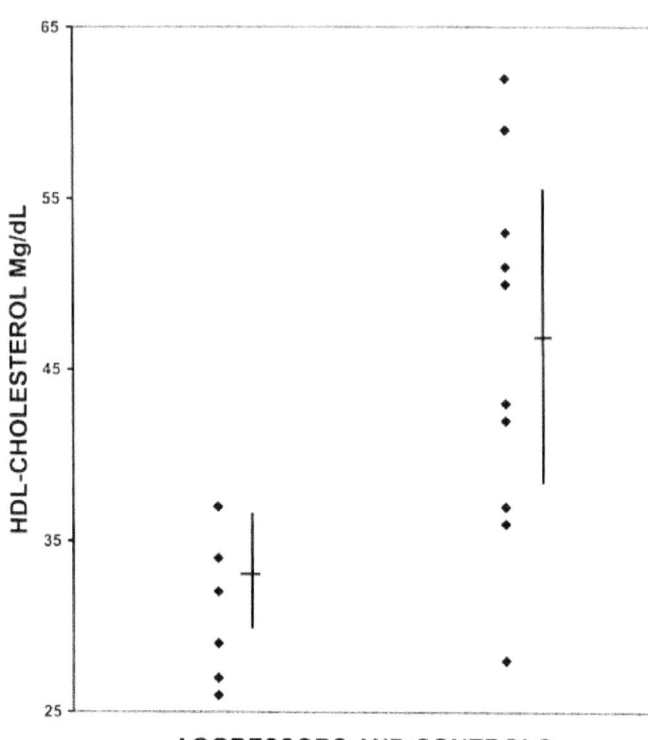

Figure: 3. Difference in the mean value of HDL-C levels between the aggressors and controls. Mean values ± one standard deviation are shown. Two tailed Exact p = 0.001. Note that despite overlap between the groups, the HDL-C level in aggressors was always less than 40 mg/dl. This difference remained significant after data were adjusted for BMI, serum triglycerides, and use of atypical psychotropic drugs.

4. Low LDL-C level, keeping HDL-C constant at less than 45 mg/dl, and BMI at less than 35, was associated with (figure: 4) assaultive behavior (p = 0.03). Unadjusted LDL-C as such did not show a significant difference in its mean values between groups.

Figure: 4
LDL-Cholesterol of Groups
(BMI ≤ 35 and HDL-C ≤ 45 mg/dL.)

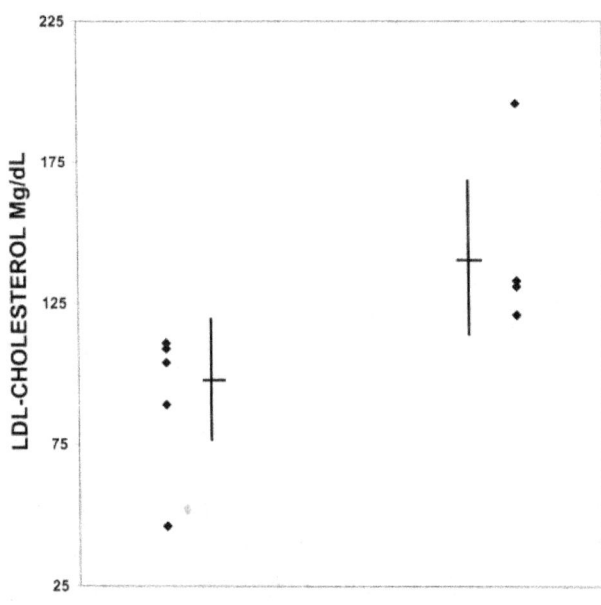

Figure: 4. Low LDL-C level, only after keeping the BMI constant at less than 35, and HDL-C at less than 45 mg/dl, was associated with aggressive behavior (p = 0.03). Unadjusted LDL-C level as such did not differ between the two groups. Mean levels ± one standard deviation are shown.

AGGRESSORS AND CONTROLS

No drug therapy or diet therapy served to distinguish the two groups. There were total 21 patients who were receiving atypical psychotropics, and 15 of them (and none others) were also receiving a low fat diet, together with gemfibrozil, atorvastatin, or pravastatin, either for primary cardiac prevention, or to counteract hyperlipidemic side effect of the atypical psychotropic drugs. Excluding these patients sharpened the results presented, without affecting their nature.

✲✲✲

DISCUSSION

An association between low blood level of total cholesterol and violence has been recently reviewed (9), but it still remains controversial whether there is any difference between "low" cholesterol and that which is "lowered" with diet and drug therapy. The importance of controlling hyperlipidemia to prevent cardiac deaths serves to sharpen the debate on the prudence of lowering lipid levels.

Although there is little doubt about the association of low cholesterol and violence in psychiatric patients (10), the potential for a possible increase in violent behavior brought about or aggravated by lowering cholesterol in these patients raises a serious dilemma. Except suicide, violence is directed at others, especially at the family members and other caregivers.

The newer so called "atypical" psychotropic drugs like clozaril, olanzapine, risperidone, quetiapine, ziprazidone, etc., are all to a greater or lesser extent associated with significant weight gain, and hyperlipidemia (8). Many drugs used to treat Human Immunodeficiency Virus (HIV) infection, common in prison inmates, also have hyperlipidemic side effects. Mood stabilizing drugs like valroic acid are also associated with significant weight gain (11).

Total cholesterol level does not yield a consistent association with violence. Our data showed no relation between total cholesterol and physically assaultive behavior (figure: 1). However, the latter was significantly associated with higher triglycerides level (figure: 2), and lower HDL-C (figure: 3).

Associations of these lipids with assaultive behavior are independent of their own mutual reciprocal relationship (see "Results"). Therefore, when these two are not separated out, their contrasting associations with physically assaultive behavior may nullify that of total cholesterol with assaultive behavior, since both these variables are components of "total" cholesterol.

Profusion of literature on total cholesterol level notwithstanding, there is a paucity of data on various lipid fractions like triglycerides, and more so on HDL-C, and LDL-C. As an explanation for the association of *high* total cholesterol with violence observed in one and the only such study (12), it was suggested that alcohol intake by the study subjects may have increased HDL-C and also increased the violent activity (13), thereby giving a spurious association of violence with high HDL-C level.

Results of studies involving psychiatric patients, regarding lipid fractions and violence give varying answers. Some have found no relation (7) of lipid profile with violence, or any difference in total cholesterol level, between patients with mania and depression, regardless of violence and suicidal behavior (14). Mean triglyceride level did differ significantly between our groups (figure: 2), but did not give a clear predictive cutoff between aggressors and controls. Patients receiving atypical psychotropic drugs and those not receiving them both showed an association between high triglycerides and assaultive behavior.

HDL-C (figure: 3) stands out as the best *post hoc* indicator of assaultive behavior. Despite overlap, no aggressor had HDL-C level higher than 40 mg/dl. Low HDL-C level provided a sharper demarkation after it was adjusted for the BMI (not shown). HDL-C level increases (15) with increasing age, alcohol intake (12), and is higher in women, while it decreases (16) with cigarette smoking, and with increasing BMI. Our groups were matched for age and sex, and patients were prohibited from drinking alcohol, according to the hospital policy.

About 75% of psychiatric inpatients are smokers (17). Our hospital was phasing out smoking to go smoke-free within two months after the study period. Patients were allowed three smoking breaks during the day during the study period. Smoking is inversely related to both, HDL-C and with BMI (16), and both the latter are inversely interrelated (see "Results"). Probably, their complex interplay had little, if any, effect on our data.

Obesity (and high BMI), either drug induced or otherwise is literally a "growing" problem. Studies aimed at settling the dilemma of whether or not to lower the lipid levels in the general population with the statins and other drugs are noted (18) to exclude psychiatric patients. Maybe, it is assumed that these patients as a group are violent, even though patients with schizophrenia have been shown to be violent only if they are noncompliant with treatments or are active drug abusers (19). Excluding psychiatric patients from such studies will only perpetuate their stereotype as being violent, and worse still, leave out the very group of individuals in whom the answer to the whole question of a relation between violence and either low or lowered lipid levels is of immediate and crucial importance.

Despite the controversy, psychiatric patients are being treated with exercise regimens, low fat diets, and lipid lowering drugs as needed to prevent or treat drug induced and other dyslipidemias. The treatment aims at lowering triglycerides and at raising HDL-C. That is exactly what wold have to be done to decrease aggressive and violent behavior, assuming for now, a cause and effect relationship between lipids and physically assaultive behavior. In short, our data do not show any reason for not preventing or not treating hyperlipidemia for the fear of increasing the violence.

There is a caveat. While low HDL-C and high triglycerides are the lipid fractions most significantly associated with aggressive behavior, low LDL-C (adjusted for BMI, and for HDL-C, figure: 4) below 115 mg/dl also showed a significant association with physically assaultive behavior ($p = 0.03$). As shown by the data presented, lowering triglycerides and raising HDL-C levels with treatment cannot explain an increase in violent deaths on lowering total cholesterol level, observed in some studies (1). Low LDL-C may be more relevant in explaining that.

We may want to question assertions like "There is nothing like a *low* cholesterol level (20)." Although normalizing lipid levels may be understandable, lowering even the LDL-C component, the so called *bad* cholesterol below normal may not be advisable in everybody. Moreover, without an established causative effect of lipids on violence, treating lipid levels as such to ameliorate physically assaultive behavior and violence is not justifiable either.

In conclusion, we have revisited the low cholesterol-violence controversy in population at large and in psychiatric patients. High triglycerides, low HDL-C, and low LDL-C are associated with physically assaultive behavior. There is no reason for not normalizing lipid levels judiciously in psychiatric patients with history of violence, and probably in the population at large as well. Lowering LDL-C below 115 mg/dl may have to be approached cautiously. Lipid levels per se are not yet recommended for their ability to predict physically assaultive behavior, which is a multi-faceted issue requiring multi-pronged and congruent approaches.

BIBLIOGRAPHY

1.   The Lipid Research Clinics Program.
     The lipid research clinics coronary primary prevention
     trial results.
     JAMA 1984,251:351-364.
2.   Randomized trial of cholesterol lowering in 4444 patients
     with coronary heart disease: the Scandinavian Simvastatin
     Survival Study.
     Lancet, 1994, 344:1383-1389.
3.   Schlinienger JL.
     The cholesterol controversy.
     Presse Med., 1995, 24:471-473.
4.   Manfredini R, Caracole S, Salmi R, Borai B, Tomalley A,
     Gallerani M.
     The association of low cholesterol with depression and
     suicidal behaviors: new hypotheses for the missing link.
     J Int Med Res, 2000,28:247-257.

5.   Golomb BA, Cirque MH, White H, Dimsdale JE.
      Conceptual foundation of the USSD statin study.
      A randomized controlled trial assessing the impact of
      statins on cognition, behavior, and biochemistry.
      Arch Intern Med, 2004,164:153-162.
6.   Mufti RM, Balon R, African CL.
      Low cholesterol and violence.
      Psychiatry Serv, 1998,49:221-224.
7.   Gray RF, Corrigan FM, Strathdee A, Skinner ER, van
      Rhijn AG, Lhorrobin DF.
      Cholesterol metabolism and violence: a study of
      individuals convicted of violent crimes.
      Neuroreport, 1993,4:754-756.
8.   Wishing DA, Body JA, Meng LR, Ballon JS, Marder SR,
      Wishing WC.
      The effects of novel antipsychotics on glucose and lipid
      levels.
      J Clin Psychiatry, 2002,63(10):856-865.
9.   Golomb BA.
      Cholesterol and violence: Is there a connection?
      Ann Intern Med, 1998:478-487.
10.   Boston PF, Dursun SM, Reveley MA.
      Cholesterol and mental disorder
      Br J Psychiatry, 1996, 169:682-689.
11.   Isojarvi JI, Tauboll E, Pakarinen AJ, van Prays J, Ratty J,
      Harbo HF, Dale PO, Fauster BC, Gjerstad L, Koivunen R,
      Knip M, Tapananien JS.
      Altered ovarian function and cardiovascular risk factors in
      valproate-treated women.
      Am J Med, 2001, 111:290-296.
12.   Tanskanen A, Vartianen E, Tuomilehto J, Viinamaki H,
      Lehtonen J, Peskier P.
      High serum cholesterol and risk of suicide.
      Am J Psychiatry, 2000,157(4):648-650.
13.   Pain M, Heineken OP, Vitamo J, Klag MJ, Manning V,
      Albanes D, Caustic GW.

HDL cholesterol and mortality in Finnish men with special reference to alcohol intake.
Circulation, 1994, 90:2909-2918.

14. Huang TL.
Serum cholesterol levels in mood disorders associated with physical violence or suicide attempts in Taiwan.
Chang Gung Med J. 2001,24:563-568.

15. Thelin A, Stiernstrom EL, Holmsberg S.
Blood lipid levels in a rural male population.
J Cardiovasc Risk. 2001,8:165-174.

16. Chi D, Nikon M, Yamamoto K.
Correlates of serum high-density lipoprotein cholesterol:
A community based study of middle aged and older men and women in Japan.
Asia Pac J Public Health. 2003,15:17-22.

17. Shah BS, Ranter H.
Anti-convulsant drugs, smoking, and body weights in psychiatric inpatients.
NY Stat J Med. 1993,93:16-17.

18. Golomb BA
(Author's reply to comments on ref # 9 above)
Annal Intern Med. 1998,129:669-670.

19. Torrey EF.
Violent behavior by individuals with serious illness.
Hops Community Psychiatry. 1994,45:653-662.

20. Nissan SE, Tusk EM, Scoenhagen P, Brown BG, Ganz P, Vogel RA, Growe T, Howard G, Cooper CJ, Broody B, Grines C, DeMaria AN.
Effect of intensive compared with moderate lipid lowering therapy on progression of coronary atherosclerosis.
A randomized controlled trial.
JAMA. 2004,291:1071-1080.

***

35. LIPID PROFILE OF VARIOUS GROUPS OF NONCONFORMING PSYCHIATRIC INPATIENTS[36]

Bharat S. Shah, M.D.

Medical Specialist

ABSTRACT

Background: As a continuation of our observation of an association between low HDL cholesterol level and aggressive behavior, we studied several groups of psychiatric patients for their lipids inpatterns.

Study details: 142 patients (including 16 women) falling under the criterion "going against the medical advice" were studied. The groups included assaultive behavior, illicit smoking in the hospital, uncontrolled diabetes, psychogenic polydipsia (uncontrollable water drinking), those with positive drug screening tests, and convicted sexual offenders. Logistic Regression analysis and ANOVA tests were done to compute the "p" values.

Results: Comparison of group means revealed characteristic lipid pattern of HDL-C in aggressors, smokers, diabetic patients, and those with polydipsia. Results were significant at $p < 0.05$, or better. Logistic Regression analysis showed an inverse relationship with one being a sexual predator.

Conclusions: These data have basic science and clinical implications.

---

[36] This paper has not been written and submitted to medical journals for publication. It appears here for the first time. It has not been presented as a structured scientific paper before this.

Citation: *Shah BS.*

           Lipid profile of various groups of nonconforming psychiatric inpatients. In

           Questions, Answers, and Exclamations from the Garage of a Clinical Researcher. P. 244 - 254, 2011 Setubandh Publications, New York.

Key Words:

           Mind body connection   Behavior problems

           Lipid Fractions   Medical psychiatry

INTRODUCTION

Association of violence with low total cholesterol level has been controversial (1), but it is generally acknowledged in special settings (2) like prisons and mental health institutions. Our own data, presented elsewhere (3) showed that low HDL Cholesterol level is a better marker for aggressive behavior.

We also found association of aggressive behavior with high triglycerides level, and we concluded that there was no contraindication to correcting the dyslipidemia in psychiatric inpatients by raising their HDL level, and lowering the triglycerides one, for cardiac primary prevention, and hence, there was no real controversy regarding the approach (3).

In as much as cholesterol is used by the body to synthesize sex hormones and other steroid hormones, it is understandable that it may affect behavior, like aggression, etc. We hypothesized that cholesterol and by extrapolation, other lipid fractions may be involved in modulating other behaviors also.

We retrospectively studied lipid profiles of psychiatric inpatients with behaviors loosely grouped under "acting against the medical advice." Our data and findings are reported here.

MATERIALS AND METHODS

We did a retrospective records review study of psychiatric inpatients of the Manhattan Psychiatric Center in New York City. All patients falling under the loosely defined criterion of "going against the medical advice," and who had had a lipid profile including total cholesterol, HDL cholesterol (HDL-C), LDL cholesterol (LDL-C), and serum triglycerides on their records, were included in the study. Records of the following groups of patients were reviewed:

1. *Aggressors*, who were reported to have physically assaulted other patients, as recorded in the Incident Reports maintained by the Risk Management department of the hospital (3). Assaults on the staff were excluded, because we intended to study only the patients.

   Victims, who were assaulted by the above group. There were many role reversals between the two categories which shared several of the characteristics. Therefore, these two categories were merged.

   Multiple Events. Many patients were involved in multiple events either as aggressors, or as victims, or both. These were also included in the Aggressors group.

2. *Smokers*. Some of these have been presented separately elsewhere in part I, and *Wound Healing Paper* (4) in part II.

   Resistant Smokers: The hospital is a smoke free facility, but scattered incidents of smoking are reported off and on. Mostly the same patients are reported repeatedly. These were included in the Smokers group.

3. *Diabetics*. Patients with diabetes mellitus, types I and II, including that induced by treatment with *atypical* psychotropic drugs like clozaril, whose blood glucose could not be controlled on regular ward, requiring them to be put on a special

Diabetes Ward providing close supervision, teaching, and special diet.

4. *Polydipsia*. Patients with psychogenic polydipsia requiring treatment on a closely monitored ward for controlling their compulsive and uncontrolled water drinking behavior and hyponatremia. Those with diabetes insipidus and secondary excessive water drinking were excluded.

5. *Drug Addicts* with positive drug screen test while in the hospital. These patients managed to smuggle illicit drugs into the facility, and were caught with a positive test for illicit drugs done periodically and at random.

6. *Sexual Criminals*. The hospital has a special ward where persons (not many of whom had a psychiatric diagnosis) with a criminal history of sexual assaults, rape, stalking, sexual murders, etc., were housed under a court order.

7. *Control Group* consisting of a convenience sample of other patients not eligible to be included in any of the above groups.

No patient was included in more than one group. If a patient qualified for two or more groups, he or she was included in the group with the smallest number of patients to avoid selection bias, and to avoid comparing a patient with himself or herself. No tests were ordered for the sole purpose of this study.

Statistical tests to compare groups by AOVA were done. Logistic Regression Analysis was done for say, *Drug Abuse Yes/No* to explore its association with various lipid fractions. In this manner, all 124 (142 minus 18, table:1 with positive drug screen) would fall under "Drug Screen - No" and make up for a small control group. The "F" and "p" values for statistical significance were computed.

OBSERVATIONS AND RESULTS

The groups did not differ significantly in their mean height, age, weight, or BMI. The table shows their characteristics.

Ser #	Group Name	# of Patients	Male	Female
1	Assaults	30	27	3
2	Smoking	27	22	5
3	Diabetes	23	18	5
4	Polydipsia	13	12	1
5	Drug Abuse	18	18	0
6	Sexual Crime	13	13	0
7	Control	18	16	2
	TOTAL	**142**	**126**	**16**

Table: 1. Patients characteristics of various groups.

Total cholesterol, and LDL cholesterol levels did not significantly differ among the groups. Serum triglycerides levels in the Smokers group was significantly higher than in the Polydipsia group (Figure: 1). The former had a mean Triglyceride level of 203.8 mg/dl, $\pm$ SD 106.2; the latter had 117.6 ± 54.7. The results were statistically significant at $p < 0.01$.

Figure: 2 shows the HDL cholesterol levels among the groups. ANOVA showed that the Assaults group had a significantly lower HDL cholesterol level than the Diabetes and the Polydipsia groups. The Mean ± SD values were respectively 37 ±9.9, 47.3 ± 10.5, and 48 ± 7.6.

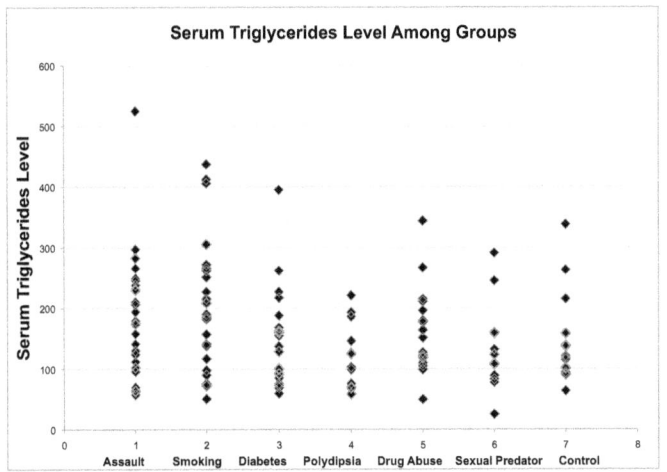

Figure: 1. Serum triglycerides levels in all seven groups are plotted. Polydipsia group (# 4) had significantly lower than the Smokers (# 2).

The Smokers (#2) also had lower HDL cholesterol than the Diabetes group (#3), and Polydipsia group, with the Mean ± SD values being 37.03 ± 10.8 for Smokers, and the rest as above. These results were significant at $p < 0.05$ or better.

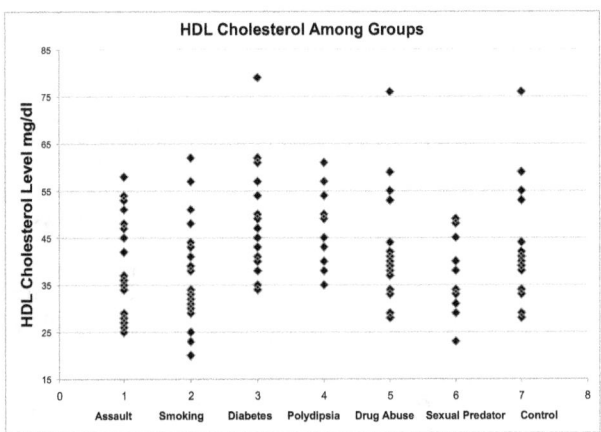

Figure: 2. HDL cholesterol level among the groups.

LDL cholesterol level differed significantly between the Diabetes group and the Polydipsia group. Mean ± SD for diabetic patients was 86.08 ± 32.5 and for the polydipsia patients it was 117.84 ± 29.15. The results were statistically significant at p <0.01.

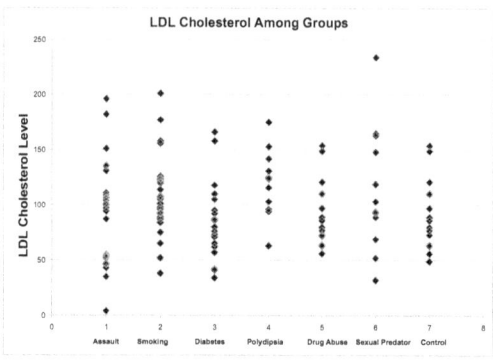

Figure: 3. LDL cholesterol among groups. The mean ± SD of LDL level in diabetic patients was significantly lower than those with polydipsia (86.08 ± 32.5 and 117.84 ± 29.15, respectively. P < 0.01).

Logistic Regression analysis showed an inverse relation between serum triglycerides and one's being a sexual predator (p = 0.028). In patients with psychogenic polydipsia, a Linear Regression analysis revealed inversely linear relation between the lowest serum sodium level recorded and the HDL-C level (not shown). The former showed (figure: 4) similar correlation with BMI (y = 109.6 +0.90x, R-squared = 0.49, r = 0.70, N = 13, p = 0.0035).

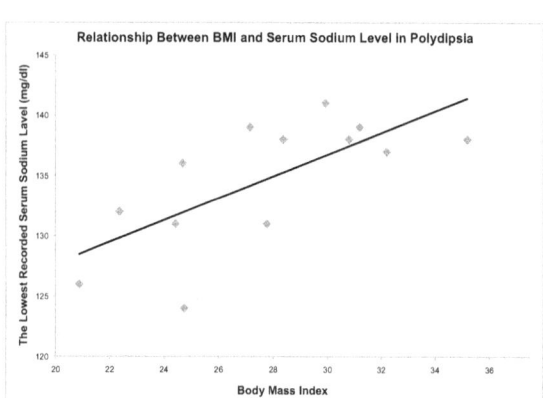

Figure: 4 shows a directly linear correlation of the Body Mass Index with the lowest recorded serum sodium level in that patient. Y = 0.9X + 109.6, R-Squared = 0.49, r = 0.7. N = 13, p = 0.0035.

Table: 2 summarizes the lipid patterns observed in four of the seven groups. These were statistically significant at p = 0.05 or better.

Groups	HDL	LDL	Triglycerides
Assault	L		
Smoking	L		H
Diabetes	H	L	
Polydipsia	H	H	L
Sexual Predators			L

Table: 2. Characteristic lipid pattern of five of the seven groups studied. Those with a positive drug screen and the control groups did not show any such pattern.

DISCUSSION

Lipids are components of sex hormones and other steroid hormones. Therefore, it is not surprising that their blood levels are associated with one or the other behavioral group. We have reported separately (3) on mutual correlations of lipid fractions, and on their correlations with age, BMI, etc.

A lower level of HDL cholesterol in the Aggressors group, as compared to the Controls has been already alluded to elsewhere in this book (3). In the present study, the Aggressors and the Victims groups were merged, and no significant difference was found in their mean HDL-C level compared to the Controls, probably thanks to dilution of data caused by merging of groups.

HDL cholesterol level was found to be significantly lower in the Aggressors group than in the Diabetes and the polydipsia groups. A relatively high, rather than low HDL level in the diabetic patients with metabolic syndrome is unexpected. The diabetes ward is a very closely monitored ward with frequent capillary blood glucose monitoring, strict diet control, and timely lipid lowering therapy, all of which may have resulted in a better HDL level. It is however, not a perfect setup, and the high HDL cholesterol level in this group does remain an enigma. The Diabetes group had more women, though (Table: 1).

Smokers have a lower HDL level (5), and despite including five women in the group, our smokers had a lower HDL-C. It is expected that they too, would show significant difference in their HDL level from patients with diabetes and polydipsia in this study. Addicted smokers in a restrictive environment may become aggressive, with or without becoming overtly assaultive, but there may be some sort of link between the two. This remains to be elucidated further.

High HDL level in the Polydipsia group came as a total surprise. Polydipsia is not reported to be accompanied by high HDL level. The latter is elevated (6) in older people and in women. The Polydipsia group had only one woman among them, and the group did not differ in its mean age from the rest. Low BMI is associated (7) with high HDL level, but BMI did not show significant difference among the groups either.

Patients with polydipsia had a higher LDL level than the smokers. This is quite interesting, since the LDL and HDL levels are expected to be reciprocal, because they are components of total cholesterol. Diabetic patients did show a relatively high HDL and low LDL levels, as one would expect mathematically. Clinically however, high LDL and low HDL are more common with diabetes and metabolic syndrome.

A negative association of triglycerides in sexual predators is of interest. Almost all psychiatric inpatients are on the atypical and other psychotropic drugs, valproic acid, etc. Which are known to elevate the triglycerides levels. The sexual predator group had generally no psychiatric diagnosis, and were not on such drugs. Our sample included all available patients, and the findings need to be verified in larger groups.

Chen et al (8) have found the total cholesterol, triglycerides, and LDL-C levels to be normal among sexual predators, and that they were lowered by Depo-provera. HDL-C was normal, and remained unchanged.

The directly linear correlation of HDL-C (p = 0.05), and the inversely linear one of the BMI with the lowest recorded serum sodium (p = 0.0035) are intriguing. HDL-C and BMI are known to be inversely related. Patients with high BMI are more likely to have increased platelets and white blood cells (9), and this may permit using a higher level of clozapine (10) that is the mainstay of treat ment of polydipsia. High BMI seems to protect against very low sodium.

Smokers also had higher triglycerides level compared to the patients with polydipsia. The latter is more intriguing than the former. Our data do not permit us to draw any conclusion about the mechanisms involved in these interesting new observations. More work is needed on larger samples to verify the findings, and to explore the factors leading to them.

In conclusion, patients who are addicted to cigarette smoking, those with diabetes mellitus type: I and II, those with polydipsia, and those who are assaultive display characteristic lipid patterns. These data have clinical and basic science implications.

BIBLIOGRAPHY

1.   Schlinienger JL.
        The cholesterol controversy.
        Presse Med., 1995, 24:471-473.
2.   Golomb BA
        (Author's reply to comments)
        Annal Intern Med. 1998,129:669-670.
3.   Shah BS.

Revisiting the cholesterol-violence controversy with new observations on various lipid fractions: A retrospective study. In
Questions, Answers, and Exclamations from the Garage of a Clinical Researcher. P. 229-243, 2011
Setubandh Publications, New York.

4. Shah BS, Foster R.
Interplay of cigarette smoking, drug abuse, season of birth, and postoperative complications. In
Questions, Answers, and Exclamations from the Garage of a Clinical Researcher. P. 206-220, 2011
Setubandh Publications, New York.

5. Brody J.
Know your numbers and improve your odds.
The New York Times, Health and Nutrition, June 28, 2005

6. Chi D, Nikon M, Yamamoto K.
Correlates of serum high-density lipoprotein cholesterol:
A community based study of middle aged and older men and women in Japan.
Asia Pac J Public Health. 2003,15:17-22.

7. Pain M, Heineken OP, Vitamo J, Klag MJ, Manning V, Albanes D, Caustic GW.
HDL cholesterol and mortality in Finnish men with special reference to alcohol intake.
Circulation, 1994, 90:2909-2918.

8. Okonofua JA, Egan BM.
Platelet and white blood cell counts are elevated in patients with the metabolic syndrome.

9. Shah BS, Foster R.
Risk factors for acute medical complications associated with clozapine treatment: A retrospective study. In
Questions, Answers, and Exclamations from the Garage of a Clinical Researcher. P. 256-271, 2011
Setubandh Publications, New York.

36. RISK FACTORS FOR ACUTE MEDICAL COMPLICATIONS ASSOCIATED WITH CLOZAPINE TREATMENT: A RETROSPECTIVE STUDY[37]

Bharat S. Shah, M.D.
Medical Specialist

Rogelio Foster, M.D.
Director of Medicine

ABSTRACT

Background: Clozapine is used in resistant cases of schizophrenia, aggression, and suicidal ideations. Its blood levels are of limited practical value in predicting complications.

Hypothesis: We hypothesized that there are patient related factors that can help us to identify high risk population. Clozapine blood level determination, adjusted for such confounding or modulating factors, may be made applicable for clinical practice.

Methods: We did a retrospective analysis of data covering an 18 month period, gathered by merging three databases, viz., on weekly white blood cell (WBC) counts, clozapine blood levels, and complications associated with clozapine therapy. Age and Body Mass Index (BMI) data were gathered from patients' records. Relationship of variables with incidence and frequency of acute medical complications (neutropenia, seizures, falls, hypotension, tachycardia) was explored. Chi-square, ANOVA, or Regression analyses were done.

Results: Including 15 women, 118 patients receiving clozapine by itself or with other drugs were studied. 70% of pa-

---

[37] From the Medical Services of Manhattan Psychiatric Center, an academic affiliation of the New York University Medical Center, New York.

tients had at least one (1-10) complication. BMI < 30, (and age > 45 years in women) were significant risk factors for developing complications. Ratio of lowest absolute neutrophil count over the highest clozapine blood level (LANC/HBLC, "the ratio") showed significant correlations with occurrence and frequency of complications, with proportion of patients with complications, with BMI and with age.

Conclusion: Risk factors for acute complications associated with clozapine therapy are identified, and a model based on the ratio LANC/HBLC is presented to help predict and possibly prevent clozapine related acute complications.

Citation: Shah BS.

   Risk factors for acute medical complications associated with clozapine treatment: A retrospective study. In

   Questions, Answers, and Exclamations from the Garage of a Clinical Researcher. P. 256 - 271, 2011 Setubandh Publications, New York.

Key Words: Hyperglycemia   Hypotension   Seizures
            Tachycardia   Ketonuria

INTRODUCTION

Clozapine has been a valuable atypical psychotropic drug for the treatment of patients with schizophrenia refractory to other drugs, especially that of aggressive, violent, and suicidal patients. It is effective in management of psychogenic polydipsia, and promising in treatment of drug addiction (1). Like other atypicals, it is less likely to cause tardive dyskinesia, and extrapyramidal symptoms. However, it can cause sedation, constipation, weight gain (2), obesity, glucose intolerance, diabetes mellitus, diabetic ketoacidosis, and can cause death.

In addition, it can cause leucopenia, especially neutropenia, and in some cases fatal agranulocytosis (3). It can induce hypertension, hypotension, severe tachycardia, and neurological complications such as myoclonic jerks, tonic-clonic seizures (4), and falls. Monitoring of clozapine blood level has been of little practical value for predicting complications, except to verify patients' compliance with therapy. Some association between clozapine level and neurological complications has been observed (5).

These severe and unpredictable complications preclude widespread use of the drug, require frequent blood drawing, and increase dropout rate from treatment (6), medical morbidity, hospitalizations, personnel costs, and mortality. The Medical Services of Manhattan Psychiatric Center undertook a retrospective, noninterventional study to explore several variables that can help one in identifying the patient group(s) at high risk, and factors associated with various types and frequency of complications, to enable us to predict, and possibly prevent the clozapine associated acute medical complications.

MATERIALS AND METHODS

Manhattan Psychiatric Center is a 350 bed inpatient psychiatric facility operated by the New York State Office of Mental Health, receiving patients from other hospitals and from the prison system. Most patients are males (75%), African Americans, with a few Hispanics and Whites. Commonest psychiatric diagnoses are schizophrenia of various types (70%), bipolar disorder (20%), major depression (10%). Personality disorders, history of illicit drug abuse and that of criminal violence are quite common.

Every ward has a psychiatrist and a medical specialist assigned to it. Complete blood count is done on all patients receiving clozapine, either weekly or every other week, according to a standard protocol. Clozapine dosage is titrated depending upon the white blood cell (WBC) count, and absolute neutrophil count (ANC). When the latter drops to 800/cmm. clozapine therapy is discontinued. Clozapine level is done periodically at the discretion of the treating psychiatrist who interprets it in the clinical context, somewhat empirically.

Cases of neutropenia not responding to clozapine withdrawal are assessed by the medical specialist. Seizures, myoclonic jerks, falls, hypotension (100/70 mm of Hg, accompanied by dizziness, weakness, etc.), hypertension, tachycardia of more than 100/ min, hyperglycemia, ketonuria, hypoglycemia, are reported every morning in hospital wide rounds, and are entered in a computer database. Sedation, inability to maintain balance and posture, newly diagnosed diabetes, etc., are not always reported as such, unless they are severe or they result in fall, seizures, and so on. Similarly, several complications recurring on the same day or within a few days may be underreported.

During the 18 month period from April 1, 2003, through September 30, 2004, 159 patients receiving clozapine had 5844 determinations of their white blood cells (WBC) count, and absolute neutrophil count. During the same period, 116 patients had 1097 determinations of their clozapine blood levels. Merging these two databases yielded data on 118 patients, including 15 women. Additional data on seizures, myoclonus and falls were obtained from the neurologist who is frequently called to see such patients not reported elsewhere.

Data on sex, date of birth, height and weight were retrieved from patients' records, and Body Mass Index (BMI) was computed according to the formula, BMI = Weight in Kg/Height in Meters squared. Complete data on BMI, clozapine level and ANC were available for 93 patients. The sexes did not differ in age (women mean age $\pm$ SD 38.5 $\pm$ 13.47, men 40.5 $\pm$ 11.06, p > 0.05). Women were significantly more obese (BMI 35.5 $\pm$ 11.6 SD as compared to 29.12 $\pm$ 7.36 SD in men, p = 0.018).

The ANC, clozapine level, and occurrence of medical complications generally did not coincide. For the final analyses, the highest blood level of clozapine (HBLC), lowest absolute neutrophil count (LANC), and BMI nearest to June 2004 were chosen, and only one row of data per patient was arrived at. Concomitant treatment with other psychoactive drugs was accepted.

Each patient was categorized as having complication – (1) "None," (2) "other" than neutropenia, (3) "Neutropenia (ANC < 3000/c. mm)," and having (4) "Both" (neutropenia plus a medical complication). These categories were non-overlapping. Frequency of complications for each patient was also computed, and it was treated as a separate dependent variable.

Statistical analyses were done using Chi-Square test, Linear Regression and Correlation, or Analysis Of Variance (ANOVA), and One-tailed Exact "p" values were computed. Patients with missing BMI, ANC, or clozapine level data were excluded from that particular part of analysis.

OBSERVATIONS AND RESULTS

Among 118 patients, there were 15 women and 103 men. Four women and 30 men (28.8% of the total) had no complications, while the remaining 84 (71.3%) had one or more complications (table: 1). The table also indicates complications categorized by type and by sex of the patient. There was no overall difference in the complication rate between the sexes. Women had relatively higher occurrence of "other" (complications without neutropenia), while men had a higher occurrence of "both" (complications in addition to neutropenia), the difference was statistically significant (One-tailed Exact p = 0.0471).

TABLE: 1. CATEGORIES OF COMPLICATIONS AND SEXES

CATEGORY	FEMALE	MALE	SUBTOTAL
1. NONE	4 (11.76%)	30 (88.23%)	34 (28.81%)
2. OTHER	5 (25%)	15 (75%)	20 (16.94%)
3. NEUTROPENIA	5 (13.15%)	33 (86.84%)	38 (32.20%)
4. BOTH	1 (3.84%)	25 (96.15%)	26 (22.03%)
TOTAL	15 (12.71%)	103 (87.28%)	118 (100%)

Table: 1. More than 70% of all patients had developed complications. Women were more likely to have complications "other" than neutropenia, while men more likely to have complications besides neutropenia ("Both," that is). This difference between men and women was statistically significant (Chi-Square Test, 2 x 2 table, Exact one-tailed p = 0.0471). Several patients had multiple complications, but each patient is included only once in only one of the non-overlapping categories in this table.

These 84 patients had suffered a total of 173 complications. Many patients had several complications. In addition to neutropenia ("Neutropenia" plus "Both" categories in table: 1) which occurred in 64 patients, other complications were: seizures and myoclonic jerks (28), falls (24), obtundation (2), hypotension (20), tachycardia (6), fever (3), ketonuria (2). All 28 episodes of myoclonic jerks or convulsive seizures took place in eight male patients, and none in female patients. Both episodes of hyperglycemia (capillary blood glucose level 300 mg/dl) with ketonuria also occurred in men. Some of these required the patient to be moved to the in-house Infirmary (16), or to an outside acute care hospital (18). No deaths occurred among these patients.

As shown in table: 2, male patients with BMI in the obese range (> 30) were significantly less likely to develop complications, in contrast to those with BMI in the lean, normal, and overweight range. On the other hand, women, rather than being affected by BMI, showed a tendency for having more complications with age > 45 years (eight out of 12 women with complications, vis a vis three younger women without any complications, Exact probability = 0.076).

TABLE: 2. COMPLICATIONS IN OBESE AND NON-OBESE MEN

COMPLICATIONS	BMI <30	BMI > 30	TOTAL
YES	46	22	68
NO	9	12	21
TOTAL	55	34	89

Table: 2. Male patients with BMI less than 30, (that is, underweight, normal and overweight, but not obese), were more likely to suffer from complications. Chi-Square 4.18 (Pearson), and Exact p = 0.04. Female patients did not show any such association between BMI and complications, but women older than 45 years had a tendency to suffer from complications. BMI and year of birth showed a directly linear correlation, with older patients having a smaller BMI (R-Square = 0.10, N = 97, p = 0.00048).

BMI was directly linearly related to year of birth (BMI = 0.2174 (year of birth in 1900s) + 16.948, R^2 = 0.1079, r = 0.3284, N = 97, p < 0.001). Correcting for BMI or for age nullified association with the other variable with complications. Neither the category nor the frequency of complications showed any linear correlation with clozapine blood level (day to day value, or mean value, or the highest value).

Highest clozapine blood level (HBLC) showed a directly linear correlation with the lowest absolute neutrophil count (LANC) in all patients, more strongly so in those who were older than 45 years, and in patients who had developed complications (not shown, Y = 614.8 + 102.43 X, r = 0.27, R^2 = 0.07, N = 74, p = 0.0084). Figure: 1 shows the isopleths of various values (0.5 through 20) of the ratio of LANC/HBLC.

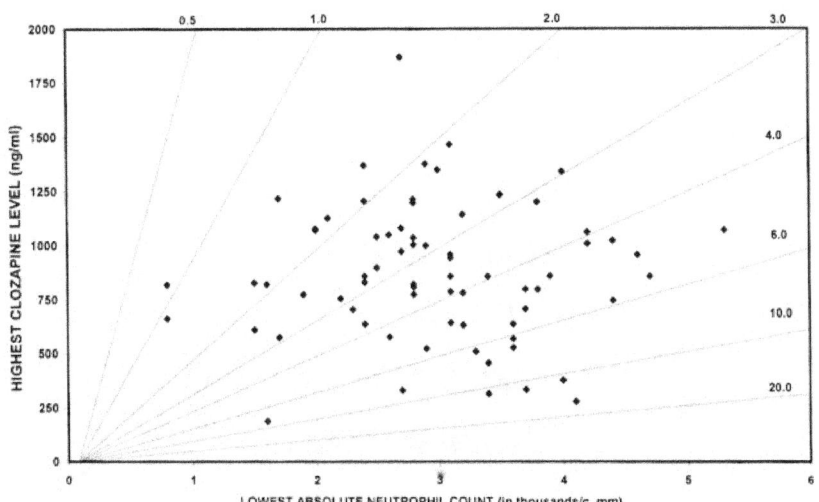

Figure: 1. This illustration shows only those patients who had developed any complication. Each data point represents one patient. Superimposed on the scattergram are the isopleths of values of the ratio LANC/HBLC, varying from 0.5 to 20. Each isopleth indicates vulnerability of the patient with that ratio to complications, as indicated by ALL data points falling below and to the right of it. For example, a patient with the ratio 20 did not have any complication, while the one with the ratio 0.5 is 100% likely to have had one. The current paper uses "four" as a practical value of the ratio for discussion.

As shown in the figure, most of the complications occurred when the ratio was between two and six. The isopleth "four" passes through the point LANC 4000/cmm and clozapine level 1000 ng/ml. It also passes through the "therapeutic" level 750 ng/ml and ANC 3000/c.mm, and hence, it is used as a practical reference point for discussion in this paper.

However, complications occurred at "four" or any other ratio between 0.5 and 20, the lower the ratio, more likely were the complications, (that is, all data points below and to the right of any particular isopleth in figure: 1).

The figure: 2 which includes patients without any complications as well, shows that when the ratio was 5-6, the number of patients with and without complications was the same. As the ratio fell to two and lower, all 17 patients had some complication. When the ratio increased to higher values, proportion of those without any complication exceeded those with complications.

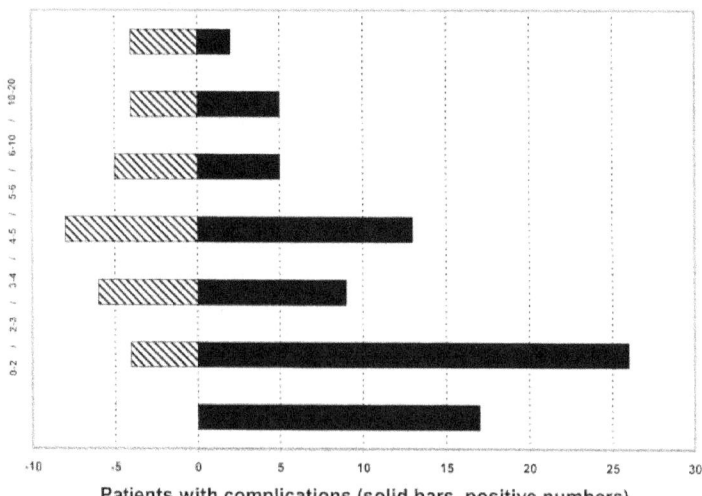

Patients with complications (solid bars, positive numbers)

Figure: 2. Proportion of patients who developed complications (as compared with those who did not), increases as the value of the ratio LANC/HBLC decreases. When the ratio is six, those with and without any complication are equally represented. With ratio value of two, all 17 patients had complications, while the proportion of those without complications exceeds those with complications at the ratio higher than ten. The negative numbers on the horizontal axis, and hatched bars indicate patients without complications, while the solid bars indicate those with complications.

The various categories or types of complications were closely related to the ratio (not shown). Patients with no complications had a very wide range of the ratio. However, those with complications with or without neutropenia had significantly lower mean value of the ratio. Overall, One Way ANOVA with four variables, was significant at $p < 0.001$.

For the significance of difference between the means $\pm$ Standard Deviation of the ratio for "None" (5.44 $\pm$ 3.0), and "Both" (2.75 $\pm$ 1.86) the "p" value was <0.01. For that of "other" (4.22 $\pm$ 1.42) and that of "Both," the level of significance was $p < 0.05$ (the former was more common in women, while the latter, in men, *vide supra*). Corresponding value for the "neutropenia" was 3.43 $\pm$ 2.27. The total number of patients in each category was None (35), other (20), Neutropenia (33), and Both (28), for a grand total: 116.

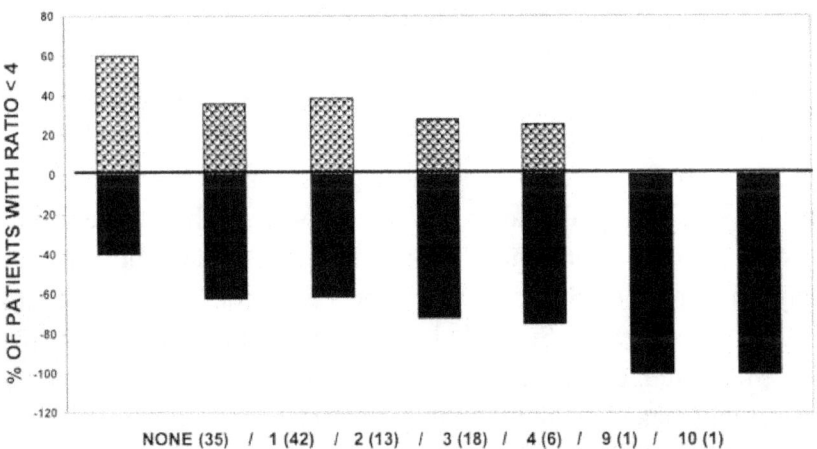

Figure: 3. This figure shows the progressive increase in the frequency of complications per patient, when proportion of patients with value of the ratio LANC/HBLC lower than four (represented here as a horizontal line at zero on the vertical axis) increases. Frequency of complications and corresponding number of patients are shown on the horizontal axis. The vertical axis shows percentage of patients in each group with the ratio > 4 (hatched bars), and with the ratio < 4 (solid bars, with negative numbers) and complications.

The ratio of the LANC/HBLC showed a close association with the frequency of complications, from none through ten, as presented in figure: 3. The horizontal line passing through the "zero" value represents the reference value of the ratio equal to "four," The horizontal axis indicates frequency of complications per patient and number of patients with that frequency in the parentheses.

The ratio showed a significant directly linear correlation (not shown) with the year of birth in 1900s, (Y = 0.091 + 0.0671X, r = 0.2792, R^2 = 0.078, N = 107, p = 0.0017). BMI also independently correlated closely with the former, with a lower value of BMI corresponding to a lower value of it (Y = 1.535 + 0.0824X, r = 0.2156, R^2 = 0.04, N = 92[38], and p = 0.0195). Lower BMI and older age both were associated with a lower value of the ratio, however, with the latter being constant at < 4, neither BMI nor age had any association with categories of complications.

DISCUSSION

Clozapine is the mainstay for treatment of resistant schizophrenia, aggression, and suicide. It is associated with numerous, serious and unpredictable complications, even when its blood level is less than therapeutic. Although, there are many factors affecting its blood level (7), the latter correlates poorly with adverse events, except in some neurological complications. Our data did not show any correlation of clozapine blood level with complications, neurological or otherwise. Several alternatives to blood level monitoring have been suggested, e.g., plasma level/dose/kg ratio, coefficient of variation (8), and even monitoring of electroencephalogram (9).

It is not implied that all adverse events were necessarily or entirely caused by clozapine. Almost all patients were receiving other psychoactive drugs as well. Despite underreporting, and con-

---

[38] Because some missing information about certain variables, the total number of patients in various tables and figures are not identical.

sidering only a limited and selected types of complications, more than 70% of patients had at least one complication. Frequency of complications varied from one to ten in these patients. In our study population, complications were more likely to occur in non-obese patients with BMI less than 30 Kg/meter squared. Female patients older than 45 years were also more prone to suffer an adverse event (p = 0.076). In our patients, BMI and age were inversely correlated, and adjusting for one variable, nullified that of the other on complications.

A directly linear correlation between HBLC and LANC came as a surprise, and provided a valuable lead for further exploration. Neutropenia caused by clozapine may compel the treating psychiatrist to lower the dosage or to discontinue the drug, thereby explaining a low level accompanying lower ANC. One can also understand a high level causally related with a lower ANC. However, explaining the association of a high LANC with a HBLC was not tenable. This led us to suspect that the drug level and the LANC may be affecting each other.

There is a case report by de Leon and Diaz (10) of an abrupt increase in clozapine blood level in presence of serious respiratory infection. Their patient's clozapine level increased to 1245 ng/ml, when the patient developed fever and pneumonia. They did not report the corresponding leucocyte count, but it was presumably high. They ascribed the rise in drug level to suppression of hepatic enzymes.

Ratio of LANC/HBLC *("the ratio" hereinafter)* correlates significantly (vide infra) with type or category of complications, frequency of complications and the relative proportion of patients with and without complications.

Clozapine blood level and ANC are routinely monitored, but have not been tied together. Clozapine affects various white blood cells, and attaches itself especially to neutrophils. We do not know whether this binding affects the effective level of the drug, and thereby decreases the incidence of complications. It appears that the LANC is somehow related to the highest level of clozapine that can be tolerated safely at that LANC. That is, the HBLC does have a bearing on complications, when taken in context of LANC.

In a short term study lasting for 12 weeks, Oyewumi et al (11) have reported weak correlations ($r < 0.20$) between clozapine blood levels and white blood cell count. Clozapine affects various white blood cells (12), and attaches itself especially to neutrophils (13). This binding may affect the effective level of the drug and thereby decrease the incidence of complications.

Okonofua reported that WBC and platelets increase in patients with the metabolic syndrome (14). This finding may explain the relationship (personal observation) of response to the atypical psychotropics and weight gain, the former being contingent upon the latter. Increased WBC and high BMI may make enable one to raise the clozapine level relatively safely.

As shown in figure: 1, patients with complications showed a similar correlation ($r = 0.27$). other patients groups, e.g., elderly patients also showed such correlations. We are dealing with highest levels and lowest neutrophil count, rather than the routine ones.

The ratio provides us with an approximate estimate of likelihood of complications (figure: 1). Although the figure: 1 shows data points of only those who did have at least one complication, this relationship between the HBLC and the LANC was observed in all patients, regardless of presence or absence of complications. In this figure, isopleths of various values of the ratio from 0.5 - 20 are overlaid. All data points to the right of and below each isopleth represent the patients who had developed complications at that, and at even higher ratios. As extreme examples, all complications are likely with the ratio 0.5, while none with the ratio 20.

We will use the ratio value "4" as a practical reference value for discussion. As can be seen from figure: 1, the "therapeutic" level of clozapine, 750 ng/ml, and LANC 3000/c.mm are on the isopleth of the ratio "4," Level of 1500 ng/ml meets the LANC 6000/c.mm, on the same isopleth. As shown in figures: 1 and 2, complications can still occur at this value (four) of the ratio. The same level 750 ng/ml, with say LANC 2000, or level 1500 with LANC 4000, will be on the isopleth of a much lower ratio, and will be more likely to be associated with complications.

Clozapine level taken together with the LANC does seem to have predictive value for complications, and it may guide the therapy. High risk patients with BMI < 30, and/or age > 45 years, may be more suitable candidates for the ratio six or higher, while younger and heavier patients may tolerate the ratio three also. Once the LANC drops under 3000/c.mm, it may not be advisable to strive to reach a therapeutic level.

Clozapine has a very narrow, if not a negative, margin of safety, since complications can occur before a therapeutic level is reached. To increase the value of the ratio, clozapine dosage may have to be lowered, or LANC may be raised by adding lithium or granulocyte colony stimulating factor, etc., hoping then to increase the dosage safely.

Except for agranulocytosis, neutropenia is generally reversible on withholding clozapine. In the present context, that amounts to raising the ratio, by decreasing its denominator. It may not be as simple. LANC, the numerator also rises. So, in figure: 1, the data point would basically move downwards and to the right, towards a higher LANC and a higher value of the ratio. The opposite can occur on giving a higher dose of clozapine.

It has been observed that by giving lithium (15), or granulocyte colony stimulating factor to elevate the LANC, clozapine therapy may be continued. Again, it may be more complex than just combating neutropenia. We may be avoiding further complications. As shown in figure: 1, even at the same clozapine level, any right shift to a higher LANC is associated with a higher ratio and fewer complications. Unlike women, men with neutropenia were ($p < 0.05$) more likely to have additional complications ("Both") than those without neutropenia,.

Besides being inversely correlated with occurrence of complications (fig: 1), and with proportion of patients who had complications (figure: 2), the ratio is related (not shown) with the type or category of complications as well. It was significantly higher in those with no complications ("None") as compared to "Both." Those with complications "other" than neutropenia, also had a significantly higher value of the ratio as compared to "Both." The former was more likely in women than in men. On the contrary, all 28 episodes of myoclonic jerks or convulsive seizures occurred in eight male patients, and none in women. Validity, mechanism, and significance of these findings need to be elucidated by further studies.

As the proportion of patients with the ratio lower than four increased (figure: 3), the frequency of complications per patient in that particular group also increased from none to 10. In the patients with more than four complications each, there were no patients with the ratio higher than four. Moreover, the other two risk factors, viz., BMI < 30, and age > 45 years (year of birth 1960 or earlier) are also associated with a lower value of the ratio. This effect disappeared, when value of the ratio was kept constant at < 4. Therefore, the association of BMI and of age with complications is probably mediated through the ratio itself.

This retrospective study can show only association, not causation. It disregards concurrent medical and psychiatric comorbidity and polypharmacy. Temporal relationship of HBLC, LANC, BMI and complications is understandably weak. Prospective studies are needed to sort out the relative importance of these three interrelated variables, *actual* blood clozapine level (BLC) and *actual* absolute neutrophil count (ANC), plus age, and to make these observations applicable to day to day clinical practice. Meanwhile, they all should receive appropriate attention.

In conclusion, the ratio LANC/HBLC is closely associated with presence of complications, their frequency, and relative proportion of those with or without complications. Thus, the ratio brings out the interdependence of HBLC, and of LANC even without neutropenia, providing a new perspective. The present study provides a new look at the old variables, viz. clozapine level, white blood cell count, age, and BMI. It offers the ratio LANC/HBLC as a new tool, together with the theoretical basis for a rational approach to clozapine therapy.

BIBLIOGRAPHY

1.   Noorsday DL, Green AI.
      Pharmacotherapy for schizophrenia and co-occurring substance use disorders. Curr Psychiatry Rep. 2003 Oct; 5(5):340-6.
2.   Wettering T.
      Bodyweight gain with antipsychotics. A comparative review.
      Drug Saf. 2001.Jan;24(1):59-73.
3.   Boshes RA, Manschreck TC, Desrosiers J, Candela S, Hanrahan-Boshes M.
      Initiation of clozapine therapy in a patient with preexisting leucopenia: a discussion of the rationale of current treatment options.
      Ann Clin Psychiatry, 2001 Dec;13(4):233-7.
4.   Lindstrom LH.
      The effect of long-term treatment with clozapine in schizophrenia: a retrospective study in 96 patients treated with clozapine for up to 13 years.
      Acta Psychiatr Scand. 1988 May;77(5):524-9.

5. Greenwood-Smith C, Lubman DI, Castle DJ.
    Serum clozapine levels: a review of their clinical utility.
    J Psychopharmacol. 2003 Jun;17(2):234-8.
6. Zito JM, Volavka J, Craig TJ, Czobor P, Banks S, Vitrai J.
    Pharmacoepidemiology of clozapine in 202 inpatients with schizophrenia.
    Ann Pharmacother. 1993 Oct;27(10);1262-9.
7. Rostami-Hodjegan A, Amin AM, Spencer EP, Lennard MS, Tucker GT, Flanagan RJ.
    Influence of dose, cigarette smoking, age, sex, and metabolic activity on plasma clozapine concentrations: a predictive model and nomograms to aid clozapine dose adjustment and to assess compliance in individual patients.
    J Clin Psychopharmacol. 2004 Feb;24(1):70-8.
8. Diaz FJ, de Leon J, Josiassen RC, Cooper TB, Simpson GM.
    Plasma clozapine concentration coefficients of variation in a long term study.
    Schizophre Res. 2005 Jan;72(2-3):131-5.
9. Gross A, Joustsiniemi SL, Rimon R, Appelberg B.
    Clozapine-induced QEEG changes correlate with clinical response in schizophrenic patients: a prospective, longitudinal study.
    Pharmacopsychiatry. 2004 May;37(3):119-22.
10. De Leon J, Diaz FJ.
    Serious respiratory infections can increase clozapine levels and contribute to side effects: a case report.
    Prog Neuropsychopharmacol Biol Psychiatry. 2003 Sept; 27(6):1059-63.
11. Hummere M, Kurz M, Barnas C, Saria A, Fleischhacker WW.
    Clozapine-induced transient white blood count disorders.
    J Clin Psychiatry. 1994 Oct; 55(10);429-32.

12.   Gardner I, Leeder JS, Chin T, Zahid N, Uetrecht JP.
       A comparison of the covalent binding of clozapine and ol-
       anzapine to human neutrophils in vitro and in vivo.
       Mol Pharmacol. 1998 Jun;53(6):999-1008.

13.   Oyewumi LK, Cernovsky ZZ, Freeman DJ, Streiner DL.
       Relation of blood counts during clozapine treatment to se-
       rum concentrations of clozapine and nor-clozapine.
       Can J Psychiatry. 2002 Dec; 47(10):977.

14.   Okonofua JA, Egan BM.
       Platelet and white blood cell counts are elevated in patients
       with the metabolic syndrome.
       J Clin Hypertens (Greenwich). 2005 dec;7(12):705-11.

15.   Patel NC, Dorson PG, Bettinger TL.
       Sudden onset of clozapine-induced agranulocytosis.
       Ann Pharmacother. 2002 Jun;36(6):1012-5.

37. GLUCOPHAGE (METFORMIN), PANIC DISORDER AND SUICIDE

(The following is reproduced from the log which I keep to clarify my thoughts and to organize them It is not addressed to anyone else, but to myself.)

Citation: *Shah BS.*
Glucophage (Metformin), panic disorder, and suicide. In
Questions, Answers, and Exclamations from the Garage of a Clinical Researcher. P. 272 - 274, 2011 Setubandh Publications, New York.

What has glucophge got to do with suicide? Nothing that we know of. There are several parts of this puzzle:

1. Panic disorder is associated with depression and suicide. These are more common in patients with agoraphobia (fear of venturing out into open spaces), who isolate themselves.

2. Infusion of sodium lactate, an alkali, precipitates panic attack very reliably in human experiments.

3. Rarely, glucophage produces lactic acidosis, especially in patients with renal, hepatic, cardiac and respiratory failures with a low oxygen level. Therefore,

4. Glucophage can, by way of lactate production, precipitate or worsen panic disorder and can lead to depression and suicidal ideations. This is what probably happened in my case[39].

---

39   See "Psychiatric Diseases, Panic Disorder, and Suicide" in part: I. Also see the information about "My Life with Panic Disorder" on the last page.

Not everything is that clear cut, except the association and temporal relationship of glucophage therapy with the events described.

1. I did not have any renal, cardiac, or respiratory problem.
2. Apparently, I did not have lactic acidosis. We will never know this and that is what a glucophage re-challenge would have told us. It may require days, weeks, or months to produce acidosis.
3. Lactate infusion produces alkalosis, with respiratory acidosis in response to it and panic attacks. This is not clear. There is secondary hyperventilation, which cannot be secondary to hypoventilation!
4. Glucophage lactic acidosis is not dose dependent and has been described in patients on 500-1500 mg daily dose, in the elderly persons.
5. Acidosis with glucophage is not always associated with high glucophage level or high lactose level. Respiratory alkalosis may occur without evident lactic acidosis.
6. Glucophage lingers in the RBCs after disappearing from plasma. The former is called the *deep compartment* and it has a longer half life.
7. Glucophage blocks the conversion of lactate to glucose in the liver. This is one way it can induce lactic acidosis.
8. Lactic acidosis may not be as rare in practice as it is in the literature. My personal physician reported to me a patient who had a low bicarbonate level (15 meq/l), which corrected itself on discontinuing glucophage.
9. Glucophage test or challenge may be potentially applied in biological diagnosis of panic disorder, if further work validates this connection.

10. Panic disorder, depression, suicidal ideations may not be sequential, but can be simultaneous aspects along a spectrum. In my case, loneliness and suicidal ideations were new phenomena, occurring despite the alprazolam therapy.
11. This connection is written up as a letter to the editor (rejected, not reproduced in here), and was reported to the FDA's Medwatch. Thank God for giving me a cool quiet head and panic attacks! Amen!

38. LONELINESS, DEPRESSION and SUICIDE

(The following is reproduced from the log which I keep to clarify my thoughts and to organize them. It is not addressed to anyone else, but to myself.)

Citation: *Shah BS.*
Loneliness, Depression, and Suicide. In
Questions, Answers, and Exclamations from the
Garage of a Clinical Researcher. P. 275 - 280, 2011
Setubandh Publications, New York.

Today I am voluntarily going to think about loneliness and depression and maybe, suicide. If loneliness is addressed, probably a major part of the other two also is taken care of. The Hindu/Jain/Buddhist scriptures and western thinkers, including Freud, I suppose, have said a lot about it.

It is a very complex subject. Let us stay at a personal level, that of my own experience[40], which in itself does not amount to much in a broader perspective. Nonetheless, the capital "I" always forms the center of the egocentric universe, no matter how much one broadens the latter.

My suicidal intrusions are gone, but I do feel loneliness as never before the episode. Glucophage (Metformin) therapy is out for the last 16-17 days now and glimipiride is in for exactly one week. I am alone most of the time. However, I notice loneliness around sundown, just before and after taking the evening dose of alprazolam (Xanax). This morning, a Saturday morning, I woke up well rested, contemplating loneliness without acutely feeling it. "Acutely" is important, because I *was* aware of it.

---

[40] See "Psychiatric Diseases, Panic Disorder, and Suicide" in part: I. Also see the information about "My Life with Panic Disorder" on the last page.

What makes loneliness *bad*? Really, nothing should. We come to this world alone and will leave it alone, as the 40th President Reagan did yesterday. Understandably, possibility and probability of my committing suicide over the last month was more important to me than death of a 93 year old, albeit a great President. I did watch most of the daylong ceremonies that the networks covered. I did not have any infatuation with death, nor did watching all that affected me in any unusual way.

In one oft-repeated comment, Mr. Reagan had said about Nancy, that there was only one person in the entire world, who can make him feel lonely, just by leaving a room full of hundreds of people. Not quoted often yet, but I have said quite a few such things about Usha, in *Sameepe*[41]. Mr. Reagan was a charming man, who had no shortage of company or activities. Yet, it took a transient absence of one person to make him feel lonely.

He was at the top by anybody's, save a super philosophical cynic's definition; and it is known to be lonely *there* at the top. You develop a teflon coating. Criticism does not stick to you, especially if you are a charming senior with a good heart and a sunny disposition, while it becomes meaningless to praise you. The only door to your inner sanctum, by way of likes and dislikes of others, is bolted shut, or even if it is left open, nobody walks through it. Then, only the *significant other* remains.

One does not have to be a Mahatma or a President or a Bill Gates to be at the top. You can reach that very easily by succeeding in the rat race for day to day things and reach a status. Shunning the status altogether, especially after being successful in the world's eyes and engaging in other important and lofty pursuits can easily put you at the top, regard-

---

[41] See the list of books on the last page.

less of how high you have climbed, since no one else is competing with you.

They may be climbing other mountains, but you are not directly aware of one another. If you succeed, there is no photographer there. If you get hurt, there is no one to apply a band aid. Most are in the valley, in the rat race, occasionally looking up to the Heavens for relief, per chance they may see you, feel praise or envy for you, but cannot convey it to you. There is no door, no lines of communication, *Mr. Jonathan Livingston Seagull* or *Jatayu*, the eagle hero of Gujarati poet Sitanshu's *Jatayu-vadh*.

One reason is, you love solitude to pursue lofty goals, to contemplate and scale new heights or depths, or to explore caverns or unpaved paths. No ordinary or average person, by definition, would even try that. You have to be different, extraordinary. Your pursuit is arduous, demanding new and different, as yet unheard of talents and skills and virtues from you, to be increasingly different from them.

But you are doing it for them anyway, aren't you? You always wanted to achieve that real success, the secret of Nirvana and offer it to the masses, who had meanwhile assumed that you were heading for the Heavens, straight from up there. You were interested in something that no one had time, desire, inclination for, or even an inkling of.

Now you saw the light and returned to the cave,[42] blinded by the darkness in the cave, you stumbled and they laughed at your ability to show them the path. *"Monsieur Lavoisier[43], the people's revolution has no use for your oxygen,"* "Mr. Socrates, here, drink your reward," and *"Mr. Christ, pick up your cross and leave the town. We will nail you down in our hearts."*

---

[42] *The Parable of the Cave*, Socrates.

[43] The French chemist, discoverer of oxygen.

Lonely are the braves! They risk or give up their lives to get something for people, the very thing that people neither want, nor seem to need, or even care for. You can only hope that people will follow your path, just as you followed that of the great men and women before you. There is no going back. The ladder was removed and used for fuel.

Thinking is dangerous. Ignorance is the most popular bliss, dependent up on mutual reinforcement, achieved by mutual praise, glorification of darkness and a total condemnation of light, even a glimmer of it. Share your thoughts and get hemlock. People do not need your oxygen, they need or at least want money. Give them what they want, or at least appear to chase money yourself, be like them for them to like you. *For you to like one another, you have to be like one another. Like does not repel the like, it attracts it.* Keep your knowledge to yourself.

I know it is not possible to turn back from solitude and lonely pursuits. The door is closed, the ladder is gone. Don't worry. People will still breathe your oxygen. They will give hemlock to you, but your thoughts will be immortal. You will die, your crucifixion will live for ever. That is why the braves die. That is why the lonely ones die. They want to be one with the masses, that is, friends and colleagues, they like to be with their likes that do not exist.

The only way for the twine to meet is in death. That is where their paths cross again, but only for a very short while, never to meet again. At that juncture, they kill you, everybody reaching your inside, or else, on your high perch, you kill yourself and in that, feel as one with them, amen!

Again coming to the practical or the applied level. Why was my loneliness more intensely felt at the twilight? The simplest answer and I believe the correct one, is that it coincides with my twice a day dosing with alprazolam for treating panic disorder. I promptly and out right reject the naive explanation that I have more company and activity during daytime. Without Nancy, Mr. Reagan felt lonely despite being amongst hundreds of people in a room bustling with action.

My feeling of loneliness is so far controlled with alprazolam, a benzodiazepine tranquilizer or an anti-anxiety drug. Panic disorder is an anxiety disorder wherein the reason for anxiety is not obvious and it may be associated with phobias or fears of places or situations.

I naively figured out earlier that loneliness can lead to suicidal ideations, suicidal thoughts and contemplation of death. It should be pointed out that the mere thought of an unwanted death can make you feel very lonely, especially when you know or find out that no psychiatrist or physician, or possibly a priest, or your spouse, or your friends can help you.

Experience shows that tranquilizers are not good in treatment of depression and suicide. That may be one more evidence to indicate that I was and am neither depressed, nor suicidal. By putting the cart before the proverbial horse, let us conclude that my loneliness was caused either by suicidal thoughts at least in part, or loneliness, or both just signified worsening of panic disorder, brought on by my taking glucophage, or by some other means.

Loneliness responding to a tranquilizer indicates its origin in anxiety and makes it accessible logically. We are not saints. We can try to claim to be selfless and dedicated whatever, but we all need and want praise, vindication, encouragement, or at least a nod. It sustains our ego (I am not a psychologist and I know hardly anything of the latter and have only a passing acquaintance with Dr. Freud's work) and its absence threatens it. Nancy walks out.

Maybe, I am addicted to being praised and am having withdrawal symptoms. Mind you, this is not a clinical and comprehensive diagnosis, but it is only a peripheral take home lesson. Although, I am a man of principles and integrity and am self-sustained, I always enjoy good company, books, music, art, history, science, etc., not to mention philosophy and humor. I am a creative person, not running after money or prestige, but there are people who are chasing them and may perceive me as a threat to their way of thinking, so dearly held by default.

Just by being different, maybe, I am becoming a threat to my colleagues, creative writers, teachers of languages, religion and culture and even without trying or despite my whole heartedly resisting, the conversation may be thrown into my lap. My friends speak highly of me among themselves, in my absence also, I know. X, Y and then Z[44] praised my writing and other things. That is scary. Fortunately, they do criticize when criticism is due.

When I say that I am self sufficient, I mean I can bear my pain and grief alone. That does not mean that I can keep the joy of discovery, the joy of probing the secrets of the universe, the wonder of life, all that to myself. I like to share all that and when people love it, I feel vindicated.

Maybe, I am inadvertently bruising some egos, who may try to keep me out of the lime light. Now one can diagnose paranoia in my case, but I am not blaming anybody else of conspiring against me. Like Ilachi Kumar[45], my efforts to please them threaten them. Well, then don't!

---

[44] Names are withheld.

[45] The hero of a Jain fable, who was son of a rich man, love-struck with the daughter of a high wire dancer who asked him to learn their art and please the king before marrying his daughter. While Ilachi is risking his life to please the king, the latter is also struck by the woman's beauty and is waiting for Ilachi Kumar to fall and die, so that he can marry her.

39. A FAMILY WITH
HBV AND HEPATIC DECOMPENSATION

Bharat S. Shah, M.D[46].

Asst. Director of Medicine.

Citation:

> *Shah BS*
>
> *A family with HBV and hepatic decompensation. In*
> *Questions, Answers, and Exclamations:*
> *From the Garage of a Clinical Researcher. P. 281-82, 2011.*
> *Setubandh Publications, New York.*

To the editor,

Thursz[47] et al, proposing a genetic basis for a persistence of hepatitis B viral (HBV) infection, did not mention observing any clustering of carriers in one or more families. Since HBV spreads easily within families, one would expect to see such clustering, especially if there is a genetic basis. One would also expect to see HBV-related hepatic decompensation in these families. A Medline literature search under the headings HBV and Family, together with Liver Failure (or Hepatic Encephalopathy) did not reveal any citation. I report here a family in which four members developed hepatic decompensation, three of whom died.

The index case is that of a woman of Asian Indian origin. Her mother, and elder brother both died of hepatic failure, the latter

---

46   From the Department of Medicine
      Woodhull Medical and Mental Health Center
      760 Broadway, Brooklyn, NY 11206.

47   Thursz MR, Kwiatkowski D, Allsopp EM, Greenwood BM,
      Thomas HC, and Hill AV.
      Association between an MHC class II allele and clearance of
      hepatitis B virus in the Gambia.
      New Engl J Med 1995; 332: 1065-9.

at age 37 years. Her remaining three brothers HBV carriers, one of whom has chronic persistent hepatitis diagnosed by a liver biopsy, Her two sisters are also HBVsAg +. Spouses of all siblings, and children who have been tested are all negative for the virus. There is no history of alcoholism, acute hepatitis, or hepatoma in the family members.

Abdominal paracentesis was negative for cancer cells. Cell count and chemistries on ascitic fluid were not done. A liver biopsy was not performed. Bone marrow biopsy showed depleted iron stores. Upper g. i. Endoscopy showed a 0.5 cm superficial ulcer in first part of the duodenum. The patient was treated with two units of packed red blood cells, sucralfate, furasimide, and spiranolactone. Her HBSAg, HBcAb, and HBeAb were positive, and the viral DNA level done two weeks after the transfusions was below detection. Ascites and edema subsided, and hemoglobin stabilized at 10.8 grams/dl.

In this family, six persons have been HBsAg positive, four of whom have had hepatic decompensation, three of the latter have died. Although several alternative explanations can be presented, *a genetic basis for susceptibility to chronic HBV infection with its complications is possible.* Since the index patient's baseline viral DNA level is not known, one can only speculate about the role of the blood transfusions (and presumably, genetically normal white cells, and CD4 lymphocytes) in clearing the viral DNA.

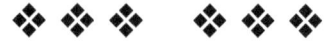

BIBLIOGRAPHY[48]
OF BHARAT S. SHAH, M.D.

1. "Mirror-Image relationship between temperature and pulse.
   JAMA 1979. 242: p. 2760.
2. Variability of body temperature — heart rate relationship induced by changes in the water balance.
   Clinical Research.1986. 34:343A.
3. Changes in the amplitude of electrocardiographic waves induced by forced water intake.
   Clinical Research. 1986. 34:343A.
4. Correction of experimental hypercapnia and hypoxemia with membrane lungs.
   ASAIO Abstracts. 1985. 14; p. 67.
5. Chemical extraction of carbon dioxide via modified peritoneal dialysis. A model simulation.
   ASAIO Abstracts. 1985. 14; p. 67.
6. A simplified extracorporeal approach to experimental ventilatory failure.
   ASAIO Journal. 1985; 223-227.
7. An in vitro model for chemical extraction of carbon dioxide via modified peritoneal dialysis.
   ASAIO Transactions. 1988; 34: 112-115.
8. Shah BS, Harold Ratner, M.D.
   Phenytoin and smoking.
   New York State J Med. 1992; 71-72.
9. Shah BS, Harold Ratner, M.D.
   Anti-convulsant drugs, smoking, and body weights in psychiatric inpatients.
   New York State J Med. 1993; 16-17.
10. Extraction of carbon dioxide via modified peritoneal dialysis.
    P. 221-27, in
    Neonatal and adult respiratory failure: Mechanisms and treatments
    Gille JP, editor
    Editions Scientifiques Elsevier (Paris), for the
    Commission of the European Communities, 1989.
11. Replacing a tracheostomy tube.
    Resident and Staff Physician. 1974. 64:318.
12. Watching the sugar with the eyes, and vice versa, in
    Questions, Answers, and Exclamations
    From the Garage of a Clinical Researcher, p. 141-145, 2011
    Setubandh Publications, New York.
13. Water induced variability of relationship between body temperature and heart rate in healthy volunteers. In
    Questions, Answers, and Exclamations from the

---

[48] The author's name is not listed if Shah is the sole writer.

Garage of a Clinical Researcher. P. 169 - 188, 2011
Setubandh Publications, New York.

14. Effect of varying oral water intake on the amplitude of electrocardiogram of healthy volunteers. In
Questions, Answers, and Exclamations from the
Garage of a Clinical Researcher. P. 189 - 205, 2011
Setubandh Publications, New York.

15. Shah BS, Foster R.
Interplay of cigarette smoking, drug abuse, season of birth, and postoperative complications. In
Questions, Answers, and Exclamations from the
Garage of a Clinical Researcher. P. 206 - 220, 2011
Setubandh Publications, New York.

16. Phenytoin, calcium channel blocking agents, and HIV infection. In
Questions, Answers, and Exclamations from the
Garage of a Clinical Researcher. P. 221 - 228, 2011
Setubandh Publications, New York.

17. Revisiting the cholesterol-violence controversy with new observations on various lipid fractions: A retrospective study. In
Questions, Answers, and Exclamations from the
Garage of a Clinical Researcher. P. 229 - 243, 2011
Setubandh Publications, New York.

18. Lipid profile of various groups of nonconforming psychiatric inpatients. In
Questions, Answers, and Exclamations from the
Garage of a Clinical Researcher. P. 244 - 254, 2011
Setubandh Publications, New York.

19. Shah BS, Foster R.
Risk factors for acute medical complications associated with clozapine treatment: A retrospective study. In
Questions, Answers, and Exclamations from the
Garage of a Clinical Researcher. P. 256 - 271, 2011
Setubandh Publications, New York.

20. Glucophage (Metformin), panic disorder, and suicide. In
Questions, Answers, and Exclamations from the
Garage of a Clinical Researcher. P. 272 - 274, 2011
Setubandh Publications, New York.

21. Loneliness, Depression, and Suicide. In
Questions, Answers, and Exclamations from the
Garage of a Clinical Researcher. P. 275 - 280, 2011
Setubandh Publications, New York.

22. A family with HBV and hepatic decompensation. In
Questions, Answers, and Exclamations:
From the Garage of a Clinical Researcher. P. 281-82, 2011.
Setubandh Publications, New York.

GLOSSARY

Since Part II is meant for readers familiar with medical terminology, terms from that part are not included in the Glossary, unless they were also used in Part I.

AAMC	Association of American Medical Colleges
ABG	arterial blood gases. Measuring oxygen and carbon dioxide level in arterial blood
Acidosis	acidemia, when the blood has more acid
Metabolic-	when the buffering capacity of the blood has decreased because of loss of bicarbonate
Respiratory-	when the acid is increased because of retention of carbon dioxide in the dissolved form
ACU	Acute care unit, a low level ICU
Ad libitum	as desired
Affiliation	The system in which unwary foreign doctors are attracted for inner city hospitals under the egis of a medical school
AIDS	Acquired Immune Deficiency Syndrome caused by the HIV
Albumin	a protein in the blood
AMA	American Medical Association, doctors' professional body
Journal of-	JAMA
Amplitude	Height of an electrical tracing
Anatomy	Study of structure of body
Anticoagulants	drugs to prevent the blood from clotting easily
Aphrodite	Goddess of beauty and sex
ASAIO	American Society for Artificial Internal Organs
Asphyxiation	choking
Atria	Receiving chambers of the heart
Attenuation	Sharpening or decrease in size or amplitude
Augmentation	increase in size or amplitude
Bad cholesterol	See "cholesterol"
BMI	Body Mass Index, weight in kg/ height in meters squared. 25 is considered normal, 25-30 overweight, and >30 is obese.
Brady	Slow, (Tachy is fast)
-cardia	Slower heart rate
Relative-	Rapid heart rate that is slower than predicted
Brahma	the creative aspect of the Hindu trinity
Bridger technic	an interim procedure done pending the decisive one
Brody's effect	Augmentation of some and attenuation of other EKG waves because of influence of conductivity of the

	intracardiac blood
Bronchus	airways below the trachea
Bronchial	pertaining to bronchus or bronchi (plural)
-toilet	cleaning the airways by suctioning (vacuuming)
Carbon dioxide	the gas produced in the body to be removed by the lungs
Dissolved-	in solution in the plasma, making the latter acidic
Buffered-	as bicarbonate which is less acidic. Blood contains 20 times as much gas in this form as it carries in the dissolved one
Cardiac output	amount of blood pumped by the heart every minute
Chlorophyll	Plant cell chemical responsible for "Photosynthesis" or using sunlight and carbon dioxide to produce starch and oxygen. It contains Magnesium instead of iron present in human hemoglobin.
Cholesterol	A fatty substance in blood, required for manufacturing sex hormones and other essential substances. When in excess, it gets deposited on the lining of arteries, including those of heart and cause a heart attack and death.
HDL-	HDL-C, high density cholesterol (more carrier protein and less fatty cholesterol), or the "good" cholesterol
LDL-	LDL-C, low density chol (more fatty cholesterol and less carrier protein), or the "bad" cholesterol
Total-	Includes HDL-C, LDL-C, and a fraction of triglycerides
Clinical years	Medical school years after completing the basic sciences or Anatomy and Physiology
CME	Continuing Medical Education for refreshing the doctors' knowledge
Complication	Something wrong that happens during the course of an operation and convalescence, e.g., infection, repeat surgery, etc.
Control group	a comparable group which is also selected with matching the age, race, sex, etc., for comparison with the experimental group.
Corporeal	pertaining to the body
Correlation	see "regression"
Dehiscence	a serious post operative complication, when a surgical abdominal wound completely opens up exposing the internal organs
Delta	$\triangle$, a Greek letter, indicates a change over a period, e.g., $\triangle BT$, means "change in body temperature" over the last hour, or another unit.
Denominator	The number below the line in a fraction
Diagnosis	Coming to conclusion about what ails a patient
Physical-	Diagnosis made based on patient's history and

	examining the living patient's body
Dialysis	Renal or kidney dialysis, filtering the blood outside the body and returning it after purifying it by removing toxins generally excreted by kidneys
Hemo-	dialysis using the blood as described above
Peritoneal-	dialysis without blood, by introducing salt solution into the abdominal cavity to remove poisons in patients with kidney failure
Modified-	peritoneal dialysis modified by the author to remove carbon dioxide
Dyslipidemia	abnormal lipid levels, see "lipidemia" hyper and hypo
Doctor	Teacher, (literally)
ECG	See EKG
ECMO	Extra-Corporeal Membrane Oxygenation, or procedure to supply oxygen by exposing the blood to oxygen across a special membrane
EEG	Electro-encephalo-gram, brain wave test
EKG	Electrocardiogram, also called EKG to avoid the confusion with EEG or the brain wave test.
-Waves	deflection or wiggles on the EKG tracing
P-	first wave, caused by electrical activity of atria or receiving chambers of the heart
QRS-	written by activity of pumping chambers or Ventricles
T-	recovery of ventricles
U-	a wave often seen after a T wave
FDA	Food and Drugs Administration, a federal watch dog agency in charge of safety and efficacy of drugs and medical devices
FMG	Foreign Medical Graduates, alien doctors, IMG or International Medical Graduates
Globulin	a protein in the blood
Good cholesterol	See "cholesterol"
Hemoglobin	Oxygen carrying protein in red blood cells, consisting of a chemical called "Heme" which contains iron, and a protein "Globin." Chlorophyll in plant cells contains Magnesium, instead of iron
Hemoresirators	a proposed term for artificial lungs used to remove carbon dioxide and provide oxygen
Heterogeneity	nonuniform or variable texture or consistency, as opposed to "Homogeneity"
HR	Heart rate, PR
HIV	Human immune-deficiency virus which causes AIDS
Homeostasis	Fixity of internal environment (*mileu interiore*), e.g., BP 120/80, temp 98.6 °F
Homogeneity	uniformity of texture or consistency, as opposed to "Heterogeneity"
Hydration	Water balance

De-	Water deficit
Voluntary-	not drinking water even when needed, unless given in one's hands
Eu-	Normal water balance
Hyper-	Excess body water
Hyper-	above, increased, more
Hypo-	below, less, decreased
ICU	Intensive care unit
IMG	see "FMG"
Impedence	resistance to passage of electrical current
Bio-	resistance caused by body
Incisional hernia	a postoperative complication in which the internal structures push through a weak surgical scar, without rupturing the latter
Indication	need, when a treatment is called for
Contra-	when a treatment is proscribed, or should not be used
Internship	First year in a hospital, after completing the medical school
Rotating-	Instead of any one branch like Surgery, to rotate through Medicine, Surgery, Pediatrics, Gynecology, etc.
Intracardiac	Within the heart
JAMA	Journal of AMA
KISS	Keep it simple, stupid!
Laxmi	Goddess of wealth
Libermeister's Rule	Mean pulse rate increases by 10 beats/sec/degree Celsius rise in body temperature.
Lipid	Fatty substances in the blood, including cholesterol and triglycerides
-emia	fat level in blood
Hyper-	increased fats
Hypo	decreased fats
-Fractions	Triglycerides, Total Cholesterol, HDL -C (high density cholesterol, or so called "good " cholesterol, and LDL-C (low density one, or the "bad" cholesterol.
M.B.B.S.	Bachelor of Medicine and Surgery (like M.D. In the USA)
Mean	average.
mileu interiore	Internal environment, its fixity is called "Homeostasis"
Mumbai	New name for Bombay, India
NIH	National Institute of Health, a research institution of Federal Government, which also provides grant sup port to outside researchers
Osmolality	concentration of salts and proteins, which determines the power of a liquid (blood, urine, etc.) to attract and

	hold water, measured in mOsmol/L (milliosmols per liter)
"p" value	a statistic indicating the probably of an observation being a chance event. Medical literature considers a 5% chance to be acceptable, that is $p \leq 0.05$
Pathology	Study of disease, or abnormal functioning of organs, as opposed to "physiology"
-gical	abnormal, diseased
Park	
Kamala Nehru-	A public park in Mumbai on the Malabar Hills
Peptic ulcer	stomach ulcer
Petri Dish	a 3" round covered glass container used to grow bacteria and other cells using a solid culture medium
pH	an indicator, called "pi-Ech" of acidity and alkalinity of a substance on a scale 0-14, Lower number indicates an acidic compound. Water is neutral, pH 7.00
Physiology	study of the working of the body systems
-ical	pertaining to Physiology, the non-diease state
Plasma	Liquid part of blood containing proteins
True-	Plasma which is not exposed to air, and which contains all its gases in the same concentration as the blood
PR	Pulse rate, HR
Psychotropics	Drugs useful in treating psychiatric diseases
Atypical-	a newer class of psychotropics that work by blocking a different kind of binding reaction
Prophylaxis	prevention
Random	Occurring by chance, not arranged, or selected
Regression	relation between two or more entities (factors, or variables) like height and weight, correlation is similar to this
Retrospective	Looking back, records review research
Saraswati	Goddess of knowledge, daughter of the creator aspect Brahma
Science	a systematic study
Basic-	Anatomy and Physiology (structure and function of body, respectively)
Seroma	Post operative complication in which 500 ml to a liter or more clear liquid collects in the wound,
Serum	Liquid part of clotted blood
Signs	objective manifestations of a disease, *symptoms* are subjective
Vital-	Temperature, pulse, respiration (TPR), plus blood pressure (BP). Inquiring about presence of pain is considered to be the *fifth vital sign*

Shock	Circulatory collapse with near zero blood pressure, extremely rapid pulse, and generally very cold skin
Statistics	Science of probability and inference
Tests	(Not included in Glossary)
Tachy	Rapid (Brady is slow)
-cardia	Rapid heart rate
Terra incognita	Unknown territory
Total Cholesterol	See "cholesterol"
TPR	Temperature, pulse, respiration,
TP-OP	BT and PR moving in *opposite* directions, MIR (Mirror Image Relationship), as opposed to TP-S, or LMR (Libermeister Relationship)
TP-S	The conventional relationship wherein body temperature (BT), and pulse (PR) both go in the *same* direction
TP-Z	BT or PR showing no (*zero*) or insignificant change, also called "Mixed" or "other"
Tracheostomy	a hole in the wind pipe to be connected to a respirator, or to be used for suctioning the secretions
Trauma	injury
Triglycerides	Fat particles in blood
Typhoid fever	A tropical infectious disease caused by bacteria, in which a *relative bradycardia* occurs, "like typhus"
Typhus	an infectious fever, meaning, "a cloud"
UPS	United Parcel Service, a private parcel and mail delivery company
Veena	a string instrument
Ventilatory deficit	amount of carbon dioxide that needs to be removed to normalize the carbon dioxide level in the blood, a proposed measure of ventilatory failure
Ventricles	pumping chambers of the heart
Vital signs	TPR, blood pressure, and pain assessment

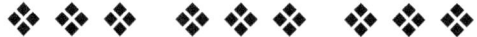

BOOKS BY BHARAT S. SHAH, M.D.

Sanskrit: An Appreciation without Apprehension
(Includes *A Crash Course to Learn the Devanagari Script*
Second edition. Our bestseller on the internet) ☆ ☆ ☆ ☆ ☆ ☆ $24

An Introduction to Jainism
(Second edition. Our bestseller on the internet) ☆ ☆ ☆ ☆ ☆ ☆ $18
(First edition, while the supplies last) $15

A Programmed Text to Learn Gujarati (Second edition) $20
A Crash Course to Learn the Gujarati Script $3

A Crash Course to Learn the Devanagari Script
(Used for Sanskrit, Hindi, and Marathi languages) $3

English for the Grandma (In Gujarati) $15

Dawn at Midnight (*A* documentary novel on awaiting
liver transplant) $12
Also available as *Kindle e-book* $8

Sameepe (A documentary popular novel,
the original version of "Dawn at Midnight," in Gujarati.
Not available on Internet. Please Email the author) $10

My Life with Panic Disorder (A documentary novel) $10
Also available as *Kindle e-book* $6

Questions, Answers, and Exclamations:
From the Garage of a Clinical Researcher
(Author's ideas for medical research being bequeathed
to the future generation.) $15

All these books are in English, unless noted otherwise. They are available from amazon.com and other internet retailers. Their detailed descriptions, cover images, sample pages, readers' reviews, comments, and shipping information, are available on website of amazon.com.

Setubandh Publications   (516) 482-6938   <bharatkumarshah@pol.net>

www.ingramcontent.com/pod-product-compliance
Lightning Source LLC
Chambersburg PA
CBHW071359170526
45165CB00001B/103